JANUA LINGUARUM

STUDIA MEMORIAE
NICOLAI VAN WIJK DEDICATA

edenda curat
C. H. VAN SCHOONEVELD
Indiana University

Series Maior, 64

THE PHYSIOLOGICAL ACTIVITY OF THE SPEECH ORGANS

An analysis of the speech-organs during the phonation of sung, spoken and whispered Czech vowels on the basis of X-ray methods

by

JANA ONDRÁČKOVÁ

1973

MOUTON

THE HAGUE · PARIS

Translated into English by D. Short

LIBRARY OF CONGRESS CATALOG CARD NUMBER: 72-94494

Printed in The Netherlands by Z.N.D., 's-Hertogenbosch.

INTRODUCTION

In recent years more and more attention has been paid to correct articulation in normal communication and in artistic speech by not only phoneticians, pedagogues and creative artists but also the wider public. We are dealing here with a wide range of problems in the complex physiological, articulatory and phonatory process, which have to be solved as a single whole on the basis of complex scientific research making use of different research methods, and in cooperation with specialists from other fields of scientific work (phoneticians, linguists, acousticians, roentgenologists, phoniatrists, pedagogues etc.).

The purpose of this work is an analysis of the articulatory relations, i.e. a phonetic study of the movements of the speech organs during the pronunciation of Czech vowels. Particular attention is paid to the articulation of sung vowels which have so far not been studied in any great detail. In singing it is above all the vocal qualities of the creative artist that are realised and evaluated; the element of communication in the majority of cases recedes into the background.[1] We find here various methods of articulation with an acoustic realisation which does not always correspond in the same way to the demands of artistic communication; i.e. it does not have the necessary esthetic effect and is not always identified in the same way by the hearer's perception.[2]

However we must not concentrate our attention only on some of the organs of articulation, and not take into account the relations of their action with the remaining speech-organs, because only by the combined action of all the organs of articulation can occur the specific conditions for the achievement of an acoustic result which will produce a specific auditory perception.[3]

[1] We often hear and read complaints about the unsatisfactory intelligibility of sung texts. On the difficulty attached to comprehensible pronunciation in German see for example H. Krech *Hochlautung und Kunstgesang*, where further literature is given (e.g. E. Fleischhauer, J. Schwierfert, R. Keldorfer, R. Morten, F. Trojan and others).

[2] Krech stresses that the vowels must preserve their character. He allows the occurrence of neutralisation only in extreme cases: "Eine Neutralisierung kann nur in hohen oder höchsten Sopranlagen gestattet sein..." (op. cit. p. 886).

[3] L. Croatto and C. Croatto-Martinolli for example express themselves very pointedly on the complexity of the articulatory process: "Le voile du palais ne peut pas être étudié comme une entité anatomique isolée ayant une fonction autonome; au contraire, il n'est qu'un des éléments variables des cavités susglottiques où, dans la parole, se modifie le son laryngien afin d'assumer des caractéristiques acoustiques déterminées que l'oreille reconnaît comme phonèmes. Son intégrité assure la

Under normal circumstances phonation is not realised without a certain acoustic effect, an effect which is the result of the perfect interplay of the physiological processes of those parts of the speech organs which participate in complicated phonation. On the surface however it appears, from the point of view of speaker and listener, as a very simple and obvious whole. And precisely because it is so obvious, and because in everyday practice we accept correct phonation and properly comprehensible articulation (we leave aside here pathological phenomena), we are very alert to deformed pronunciation of sounds as occurs for instance in bel canto. Everyone well knows that such a deformation occurs. As early as 1911 attention was drawn to it by L. Hermann.[4] This very important question has not so far been adequately studied.

Owing to the number of problems so far unsolved[5] – this work and its set problems is the first carried out for Czech – it was necessary to concentrate on the vowels, and of these only long vowels í, é, á, ó, ú spoken, sung and whispered.[6]

There are various opinions on the significance of the vowels and consonants for the intelligibility of a sung text.[7] Some authors believe that the greatest barrier to intelligibility in song are actually the consonants and that it depends on the skill of the singer to get over them quickly in order to concentrate the full value of the tone on the vowels. If correct pronunciation of the vowels gave the singer no trouble we would not hear switching of vowels so frequently.

In our research of the articulatory action of the speech-organs we used sets of various measuring apparatuses and complex phonetic methods to discover at one and the same time the articulatory relations and the acoustic form of the sounds. The machines for making parallel records were always perfectly synchronised.

In collecting material for this work we had to elaborate new research methods and

---

réalisation correcte des phénomènes normaux d'articulation et de résonance, et l'importance qu'il revêt dans ensemble de ces mécanismes s'avère évidente si, pour une raison pathologique quelconque, il ne réussit plus à remplir sa fonction."

"Physiopathologie du voile du palais", *F Ph* 11, 124-166 (1959).

4 L. Hermann, "Neue Beiträge zur Lehre von den Vokalen und ihrer Entstehung" (*Pflüger's Archiv für die gesamte Physiologie* 141, [1911] 18). Quoted after B. Hála, *Akustická podstata samohlásek*, Praha, 1941, p. 170.

5 For example R. Husson has spent a number of years working on an investigation of singer's voice and articulation in singing.

6 For a singer neither an isolated syllable nor an isolated vowel is so unusual as for a speaker. Even in the only description so far in existence of Czech spoken vowels according to roentgenograms (B. Polland – B. Hála, *Artikulace českých zvuků v roentgenových obrazech* [skiagramech], Praha 1926), it was necessary to commence with the articulation of spoken 'sustained vowels' in view of the necessarily long exposure times in those days.

7 H. Krech gives some interesting opinions on the role of the vowels in the intelligibility of a sung text. He quotes for example also the opinions of A. Honegger and R. Strauss. A. Honegger (*Ich bin Komponist*, Zürich 1952) says: "In der klassischen Gesangskunst, im Reiche des Belcanto, war der Vokal der Herrscher, denn auf A – E – I – O – U kann man den Ton so lange halten, als man nur will. Heute schleudern in einer dramatischen Deklamation die Konsonanten das Wort in den Saal, sie hämmern es." (quoted from Krech's op. cit. p. 885).

check their reliability; only partial use was made of the methods adapted to phonetic purposes.

Particularly time-absorbing was the testing and evaluating of the various contrast preparations which have been used hitherto. This finally led us to cooperation with MUDr. R. Poch with whom we found and tried in practice a method which does not require the application of any artificial contrast media i.e. no interference with the completely natural articulation of the person being studied.

As the basic method for the study of articulatory relations we again applied X-ray and cineradiographic methods without using any artificial contrast media.

Right at the beginning of our study we were aware of the complexity of the physiological process of articulation and phonation and we tried to conceive them as a whole. This effort gradually led us through serial roentgenography to cineradiographic sound recordings.

It is our pleasant duty to acknowledge our gratitude for the valuable advice and suggestions offered us during the course of the work by Academician Prof. B. Havránek, Prof. Dr. B. Hála Dr.Sc., Prof. Dr. M. Romportl Dr.Sc., Doc. Dr. F. Daneš Dr.Sc., Doc. Dr. P. Janota C.Sc., MUDr. J. Bret, Prof. Dr. A. Sychra, Dr.Sc. and MUDr. J. Kiml, C.Sc.

We are deeply obliged to Doc. MUDr. R. Poch C.Sc. for his willing aid on all sides with the X-ray work. We also received the kind assistance of the scientific workers of Humboldt University in Berlin, above all of Prof. Dr. med. W. Porstmann.

For their time-demanding cooperation we thank all those who made our research possible by acting as study-subjects, and finally we thank all others who have helped in any way in the more than ten years strenuous work on the present problem.

Last but not least I express my best thanks to my husband for his devoted aid and admirable patience.

CONTENTS

ABBREVIATIONS OF PERIODICALS

AJR	– The American Journal of Roentgenology, Radium Therapy and Nuclear Medicine
ALR	– Archiv für Laryngologie und Rhinolaryngologie
ANPE	– Archives néerlandaises de phonétique expérimentale
AO	– Archives of Otolaryngology
APPhL	– Aktuelle Probleme der Phoniatrie und Logopädie
AR	– Acta Radiologica
ARS	– Acta Radiologica Scandinavica
AUC	– Acta Universitatis Carolinae
AZ	– Akustische Zeitschrift
ČLČ	– Časopis lékařů českých
ČR	– Československá rentgenologie
FGR	– Fortschritte auf dem Gebiete der Röntgenstrahlen
FPh	– Folia phoniatrica
IJR	– The Indian Journal of Radiology
JASA	– The Journal of the Acoustical Society of America
JSHD	– Journal of Speech and Hearing Disorders
JSHR	– Journal of Speech and Hearing Research
MM	– Medizinisch-pädagogische Monatschrift für die gesamte Sprachheilkunde
NŘ	– Naše řeč
Ph	– Phonetica
R	– Radiology
SaS	– Slovo a slovesnost
SO	– Slaboproudý obzor
STL-QPSR	– Speech Transmission Laboratory – Quarterly Progress and Status Report
UCPMPh	– University of California Publications in Modern Philology
WZ	– Wissenschaftliche Zeitschrift der Martin-Luther-Universität
ZEPh	– Zeitschrift für experimentelle Phonetik
ZPhS	– Zeitschrift für Phonetik und allgemeine Sprachwissenschaft
ZPhSK	– Zeitschrift für Phonetik, Sprachwissenschaft und Kommunikationsforschung

OTHER ABBREVIATIONS

ČSAV	– Československá akademie věd /Czechoslovak Academy of Sciences/
p	– plane film
rs	– serial roentgenogram
s	– modified stereoscopic method
M	– spoken vowel
Š	– whispered vowel
Z	– sung vowel
pp, mf, ff	– pianissimo, mezzoforte, fortissimo

RA, JD, MD, JH, RJ, AM, VM, MN, HŠ, LŠ, RV – test persons

I

X-RAY METHODS

For the study of the articulatory relations in the supraglottal cavities when long Czech vowels are spoken, sung[1] and whispered we had to look for the most suitable procedures. In a series of experiments lasting more than five years we tried out many methods whose application we could assume would enable us to find the most appropriate media for our purpose[2] and a special approach for the study of articulation in its complexity.

For the complex study of the mechanisms of articulation of the speech-organs we used above all X-ray methods.

We used plane films and in addition modified stereoscopic methods with parallel sound and oscilloscope recordings.[3] Experimentally we also used tomography. A large number of pictures were obtained by serial roentgenography. Finally we made a cineradiographic sound film in three parts and two colour sound films.[4]

We concentrated great attention on searching for the most suitable methods of studying the movement and action of the tongue, the soft palate and the back wall of the throat during phonation. At the same time we had to pay attention to the acoustic side. By way of quality check of the vowels realized we verified and evaluated them according to the auditory action on the listener. Therefore we always took side

1 The importance of the scientific investigation of singing was demonstrated at the first Czechoslovak Conference on the Training of Singing Personnel by Scientific Methods, which was organised in 1955 by the Ministry of Culture and the Concert Artists Section of the Union of Czechoslovak Composers. J. Ondráčková's report of the conference is printed in *NŘ* 39 (1956) 107-108. In 1954 a commission for the scientific investigation of singing was established at the Phonetics Laboratory of the Institute of Czech Language, Czechoslovak Academy of Sciences.

2 For example the method of filming the labial aperture (P. Janota – L. Švestková, "K metodice výzkumu retní činnosti", *AUC*, Philologica supplement 1959, p. 37-44).

3 With a suitably adapted X-ray apparatus for taking two shots at an interval of 0.5 sec. with shifting of the X-ray tube of 62mm. (See also note 11, chapter 2).

4 See Price-list of Czechoslovak Scientific Films, Czechoslovak Scientific Film Association, Praha 1967:

a. "The movement of the tongue and the soft palate in the singing of vowels" (X-ray sound film), Praha – Berlin 1959/1960.
b. "Activity of the soft palate during phonation – direct shots" (colour sound film), Praha 1960.
c. "Articulatory movements of the tongue and the soft palate – direct shots" (colour sound film), Praha 1961.

by side with the X-ray picture synchronised sound recordings or even oscilloscope records.

The use of supervoltage roentgenography[5] and rotational cinefluorography[6] techniques will give promising results, but unfortunately we did not have the necessary apparatus at our disposal. Supervoltage roentgenography allows the further shortening of exposure times. It has the additional advantage that bone shadows come out faintly so that the structures of the soft parts stand out correspondingly more clearly. Rotational cinefluorography shows spatial relations by rotation of the object; in this way we obtain a three dimensional X-ray picture. While the X-ray pictures used so far give only a flat surface profile, rotational cinefluorography gives information about the spatial distribution of the articulatory organs. This is very necessary as the flat profile X-ray pictures may show the same contour of the tongue when it is simply arched, and when it is arched but with simultaneous grooving of the crest and raising of the outer edges. We found this for example with a slight departure from the absolutely central position. In such cases there appeared a double contour of the edges of the tongue.

1. THE PLANE FILM METHOD

This method has been hitherto very widely used in phonetic research. In the Prague phonetic school first use was made of it for the study of the articulation of Czech sounds in 1926 by B. Hála and B. Polland, – later by J. Chlumský, M. Romportl, K. Ohnesorg, A. Skaličková and others. This method has also been widely used abroad.[7]

The first plane X-ray films for our research, i.e. static lateral film capturing the whole area of the supraglottal cavities were obtained at the beginning of 1955 at the Institute of Clinical Physiology[8] in Prague with the cooperation of M. Romportl. The methods standard at that Institute were used during the exposure of the films: the phonation of the study subjects was checked by ear only and the exposure was

5 G. M. McDonnel, H. L. Berman, E. A. Lodmell, "Supervoltage Roentgenography", *AJR* 79 (1958) 306-320.

6 F. S. Winter, J. S. Lehmann, "Rotational cinefluorography", *AJR* 82 (1959) 120-124.

7 B. Polland – B. Hála, op. cit.; J. Chlumský, A. Pauphilet, B. Polland, *Radiografie francouzských samohlásek a polosamohlásek*, Praha 1938; M. Romportl, "Fonetická studie o ruském ы", *Slavia* 22 (1953) 529-556; K. Ohnesorg – O. Švarný, "Études expérimentales des articulations chinoises", *ČSAV* Rozpravy 65, No. 5 1955; A. Skaličková, "The Korean Vowels", *A* 23 (1955). In foreign literature there is for example L. Hegedüs, "Roentgenaufnahmen von ungarischen Vokalen", *ANPE* 13 (1937) 72-77. Hegedüs on the basis of a comparison of Russell's and Gutzmann's X-ray pictures proves that the same vowels of different languages are formed and characterised by the same position of the articulatory organs. Further: H. Koneczna – W. Zawadowski, *Obrazy rentgenograficzne głosek rosyjskich*, Warszawa 1956; N. I. Žinkin, *Mechanizmy reči*, Moskva 1958; H. H. Wängler, *Atlas deutscher Sprachlaute*, Berlin 1961, and others.

8 With the kind permission of Prof. MUDr. J. Skládal.

taken at the so called "culminatory phase" of phonation. In this way were acquired plane X-ray lateral pictures of the lips, the tongue, the soft palate, the back wall of the throat, the epiglottis and the angle of the jaws. As contrast medium was used barium paste with which were smeared the lips, tongue and soft palate of the study subject.

Later we made X-ray pictures without using any artificial contrast medium, (see chapter II – contrast media) in cooperation with the roentgenologist MUDr. R. Poch of the First Internal Clinic of the Faculty of Hygiene-Medicine of Charles' University.[9]

In view of the necessary demands of the study of the physiological activity of the speech-organs this method of static pictures was found to be inadequate. Therefore we made an earnest search for more suitable methods.

2. MODIFIED STEREOSCOPIC METHOD

In detailed analyses of X-ray films we often discovered that the speech-organs had not been caught at the "culminatory phase" of the phonation of the vowel under study, i.e. at the phase of the "proper articulation".[10] Therefore we endeavoured to overcome this weakness by making two exposures in the manner of stereoscopic photographs. We then looked at the pictures as slides with a device for looking at stereoscopic shots.[11] The plastic picture of the supraglottal cavities made it much easier to decide whether there was velopharyngeal closure during phonation.

In using X-ray methods for phonetic purposes it is very useful to apply the advantages of stereoscopic pictures which very much simplify analysis of the articulatory phase of the speech-organs.

3. THE METHOD OF SERIAL ROENTGENOGRAPHY

Both the methods described allow of only a static portrayal of the soft parts of the speech-organs in the oral and nasal-pharyngeal cavities.

Because during phonation the articulatory position of the speech-organs is not static and unchanging we tried to obtain the longest possible series of shots catching gradually the phases of articulation of the individual sounds. Under these conditions

9 With the Siemens-Heliofos we obtained altogether 106 plane films from which 70 were taken for test purposes. We employed Agfa X-ray film.

10 We use the terms on-glide, proper articulation and off-glide in the same sense as E. Dieth the terms *Anglitt*, *Klarphase* and *Abglitt* (*Vademekum der Phonetik*, Bern 1950, p. 225) and O. von Essen the terms *Anglitt*, *Mittelphase* and *Abglitt* (*Allgemeine und angewandte Phonetik*, Berlin, 1953, p. 58). We use them even for the vowels.

11 We used this method from July 1955 for 314 shots made by the Siemens-Heliofos machine on Foma film with a distance of 1 metre from the tube of the test subject and at 20 mAs.

in 1957 it was a great contribution for our work that for photographing the activity of the speech-organs during phonation we used serial roentgenography.[12]

This was the first use of this method in our phonetic research. We always photographed without artificial contrast media.

Serial roentgenography allowed us to take a series of shots in one second (4-12). Photographing began with the speech-organs having no phonation and with the mouth closed. In the series of shots were gradually recorded the speech-organs in on-glide, proper articulation and off-glide of the vowel and again the speech-organs without phonation.[13] Simultaneously and synchronously we recorded the phonated sounds on tape so that we could at any later date carry out an interpretation by confronting the individual serial roentgenograms with the sound character of the phonated vowel and relate pitch and intensity.[14]

Serial roentgenography allows us to study in picture form the mobility of the individual articulatory phases of the speech-organs. The pictures give us a very clear idea of the natural movements of the organs of articulation. From this point of view serial roentgenography represents a significant improvement against the static pictures of the speech-organs at the moment of their "culminatory articulatory phase".[15]

The advantages of serial roentgenography are particularly manifest in the study of certain special questions. Serial roentgenograms have helped to explain for example why there were significant differences in the formation of the velopharyngeal closure in the same vowel and the same person,[16] which was observed both on the plane films and on those used in the modified stereoscopic method.

On serial roentgenograms capturing syllables we can observe by studying the very

[12] The use of serial roentgenography for the study of the articulatory formation of the speech-organs has been described in the article by J. Ondráčková and R. Poch: "Zur Methodik der Untersuchung der Vokalartikulation beim Gesang", *ZPhS* 10 (1957) 258-268.

[13] On the Elema machine we took four 30cm × 30cm pictures a second on a continuous film strip. The picture obtained was somewhat enlarged as the construction of the seriograph does not allow the test subject to be right up against the cassette as is the case with plane films. The format of the picture has the advantage that it allows of precise observations and distinctions of details.

[14] For a closer explanation see the chapter on the complex recording method.

[15] By this of course we do not mean to exclude the application of the current static X-ray methods.

[16] Attempts at examining the question of the complete or incomplete velopharyngeal closure in articulation of vowels are already of an earlier date, though the possibilities available at that time could not give satisfactory results. B. Hála discovered as early as 1926 differences in the position of the soft parts of the speech-organs during articulation of the vowel *é*. On one picture of the articulatory position of the speech-organs during phonation of the vowel *é* he found there was velopharyngeal closure, whereas on another photograph of the vowel *é* articulated by the same person there was no such closure. B. Hála explains this by a nasal colouring of the second *é*. Serial roentgenograms which we have obtained during the phonation of the vowel *é* show a quite definite fluctuation of the velopharyngeal closure during phonation, although this fluctuation is not perceived as any nasal colouring of the vowel by Czech listeners.

L. Croatto and C. Croatto-Martinolli write about this in their work quoted above.

Serial roentgenography confirms the earlier supposition that not even in the articulation of non-nasal vowels is the velopharyngeal closure always firm. On the methods of expressing the degree of nasality work is being carried out for example at Halle (Institut für Sprechkunde und phonetische Sammlung) and at many other places.

rich pictorial material[17] certain transitional phenomena between the individual sounds.

Even at a frequency of 4-12 frames per second this method of serial roentgenography without the use of any artificial contrast media shows very clearly the combined action of the speech-organs, and well allows us to observe the all articulatory phases of the vowel and the means by which it is joined to the preceding consonant.

It is quite clear that to produce better conditions for the study of the MOVEMENT of the speech organs during phonation we need a greater rate per second of frames. Only cineradiography can give us a real record of the movements of the speech organs.

4. THE CINERADIOGRAPHIC METHOD

In isolated instances experiments have been carried out to photograph directly the fluorescent screen picture.[18] However cineradiography came up against quite significant technical difficulties. It was impossible to obtain sufficiently clear-cut X-ray pictures; nor was it possible to take an adequate number pictures per second so that when projected they gave a natural picture of the smooth movement of the speech-organs. Neither a distinct image amplification and an improvement of the object lenses, not an increase in the sensitivity of the films designed for a fluorescent screen picture brought for a long time complete satisfaction. As long as it remained possible to make only 8 to 12 exposures a second, it was necessary to duplicate each picture in the copy to give at least partially the impression of smooth movement. However the films acquired by this method are not sufficiently sharp and the movements of the speech-organs are so fast that it is impossible to use the films for more detailed analyses.

Very recently there have been constructed efficient electronic image amplifiers. By an increase in the brightness of the fluorescent screen picture, exposure time is sharply cut which allows of absolutely natural filming of the smooth movement of the speech-organs during phonation.[19]

[17] At the radiological clinic in Hradec Králové by the method of serial roentgenography there have been obtained 104 films of the sung syllables *bí, bé, bá, bó, bú* realised by male and female voices. Further seriograms were obtained in the X-ray department of the Hospital in Praha-Střešovice (400 seriograms at an average frequency of 4 pictures per second). We were again working with the machine Elema at 14 mAs. The films show the sung and spoken syllables *bí, bé, bá, bó, bú* in their realisations by four persons (two women and two men). By way of cooperation with the Theatrical Institute of the Ministry of Education we obtained a further 300 films recording the speech-organs during the singing of an excerpt of a song.

[18] For example H. Gutzman whose film was shown in Prague at the fourth Congress of Phoniatrics and Logopedics in 1930. M. Romportl in 1956 also made an attempt to record the movements of the speech organs during the articulation of Czech words at a frequency of 18 shots per second.

[19] Cineradiographic recordings for the study of the speech-organs in the supraglottal cavities in normal and pathological subjects were used for example in 1959 by L. Croatto and C. Croatto-Martinolli. They reproduce a specimen from their film in the work quoted. In 1959 there also ap-

There already exists a number of high quality cineradiographic films of the movements of the speech-organs; in the majority of cases however use is still made of artificial contrast media.

After many years of experience gained in analysing several hundred static X-ray pictures it has been confirmed that it is quite essential to use above all cineradiographic methods for the study of the movements of the articulatory organs during NORMAL phonation.

In cooperation with the Institute for Roentgenology and Radiology of Charité in Berlin we have acquired a suitable X-ray apparatus with a sufficiently efficient image amplifier for making cineradiographic recordings. In 1959 at that Institute we made three cineradiographic X-ray films. These are the first pictures of the articulatory movements of the speech-organs during the phonation of Czech spoken, sung and whispered vowels, isolated and in syllables, at different pitch with the same intensity, and at the same pitch with different intensity and realised by three singers of repute.[20]

The cineradiographic method with the use of an image amplifier has allowed us to obtain the most suitable material so far for analyses of the action of the speech-organs in the supraglottal cavities in conditions of their normal movement and without the use of artificial contrast media. It is an absolutely essential and so far the most adequate method for the study of the physiological and pathological action of the articulatory and phonatory organs.

---

peared the study by A. Sovijärvi. The author remarks the influence of consonants on the vowels *a* and *i*. ("Über die Veränderlichkeit der Zungestellung und der entsprechenden akustischen Schwankungsgebiete der Vokale auf Grund eines Röntgentonfilms gesprochener finnischer Sätze", *Phonetica* 1959, supplement to Vol. 4.).

The authors, A. Mitrinowicz-Modrzejewska and St. Kruszewski ("Röntgenkinematographie und die Pathologie der Stimme", *FPh* 13 [1961] 164-173), highlight the significance of cineradiography for the study of vowels, for the treatment of cleft palate, for phonetics and phoniatrics. They however make use of contrast media which they introduce via the nasal and not the oral cavity in their examinations. During cineradiographic filming the person being examined speaks or sings freely without being hampered by the device introduced into the oral cavity or the larynx. This is particularly important in the examination of singers and actors.

20 See the report "První rentgenokinematografický záznam z oblasti fonetiky češtiny", *Bulletin of ČSAV* 5 (1959) 8; in more detail see J. Ondráčková, "První rentgenokinematografický záznam artikulace českých zpívaných vokálů", *ČSAV* Věstník 69 (1960) 125-126, J. Ondráčková – R. Poch, Nativní rentgenokinematografie mluvidel, ČR 16 (1962) 92-99, J. Ondráčková – R. Poch, "New roentgenographic methods in the research of the activity of the articulatory organs", *IJR* 16 (1962) 137-150, and J. Ondráčková, "The movement of the tongue and the soft palate in the singing of vowels", *FPh* 13 (1961) 99-106.

In the recording of the three parts of this cineradiographic film in Berlin in 1959 we received the very willing aid particularly of Prof. MUDr. W. Porstmann, J. Kyritz, and Prof. MUDr. G. Burgemeister. The necessary apparatus was loaned by the Phonetics Institute of Humboldt University in Berlin.

The sound film with the commentary was projected at the International Congress of the Association for Scientific Films in Prague in 1960, at the IVth International Congress for Phonetic Sciences in Helsinki in 1961, in 1962 at the International Scientific film Congress in Sydney, at the XIIth International Congress for Logopedics and Phoniatrics in Padua, and at the XIVth International Congress of the Association for Scientific Films in Warsaw. It is kept in the Film library of ČSAV in Prague.

Technical progress allows us to use this method on a wide scale; cineradiographic recordings taken with higher frequency of pictures p.s. enable us for example to study the movements of the speech-organs even when the movement is slowed down in a natural way without extraneous influence.

5. THE TOMOGRAPHIC METHOD

Tomography was used only experimentally in our research.

For example L. Croatto and C. Croatto-Martinolli applied the tomographic method in their study of the function of the soft palate from the phoniatric point of view. Their tomograms included the movements of the side walls of the pharynx in the frontal projection as possible compensatory movements in the case of the incomplete closure of the soft palate.

We think that all the above-mentioned X-ray methods are suitable for phonetic purposes in various complementary combinations.

II

METHODOLOGICAL PROBLEMS SOLVED

While working out and evaluating new methods and researching for the most suitable study material, we had to solve several intermediate problems. The main one was the question of the use of contrast media. Then we had to work out a method of complex recording, to attempt to find a method for objectively measuring the X-ray pictures, and a method for the comparative evaluation of individual film frames.

1. CONTRAST MEDIA

X-ray methods applied for phonetic research are not a new idea, but they have never been without difficulties from the beginning. One major complication is the fact that for an articulatory picture of the speech-organs during phonation the movement of the soft parts of the organs is very relevant and these of course are by no means as clearly visible on X-ray pictures as the hard parts of the same organs. Therefore it was not easy to obtain sufficiently clear X-ray pictures of the soft parts of the speech organs, and researchers for a long period tried to find a good way of bringing out the contours of the lips, tongue, soft palate and the back wall of the throat. It is a matter of some surprise that for the study of the action of such fine organs as the articulatory mechanism some quite rough methods have been used which are not without influence on the PHYSIOLOGICAL action of the speech organs.[1]

[1] A review of the older such attempts is to be found in the quoted publication of B. Polland and B. Hála, *Artikulace českých zvuků v roentgenových obrazech* (skiagramech), Prague 1926, where are critically evaluated the contrast media and solid objects used. Mention is made of the unsuitability of some methods by B. Hála also in his review of the work of J. Chlumský, B. Polland and A. Pauphilet, "Radiografie francouzských samohlásek a polosamohlásek", *ČMF* 27, 1941, 394 n. "Both" (i.e. the American Russel and the German phoniatrician Gutzmann the younger) "covered the tongue with a fine skin which is used in gilding and by it spread barium sulphate on the tongue... only the skin – as Gutzmann discovered – often rolls up and one patient even swallowed it. In addition to this method they also tried iodipine injections though these caused pain to the test subjects and are therefore unsuitable." J. Chlumský in the above mentioned work writes on page 35: "At the end of the description of French *a* we must touch on one more matter of dispute, to wit the position of the soft palate during the pronunciation of *a*. Purkyně's pupil J. Czermák found from his very basic but interesting experiments that with all vowels the soft palate closes the nasal passage, though with *a* it is lowest and the closure weaker. Czermák used a wire to discover if there was a closure or not and

Working on the assumption that during X-ray studies of the soft parts of the speech-organs it is not possible to avoid artificial means of emphasising their contours, various contrast media were regularly used. Most frequently applied was barium, in a central stripe on the upper and lower lips, on the crest of the tongue and on the soft palate as far as the uvula; the barium could be applied to the back wall of the throat by swallowing.

In cooperation with the roentgenologist MUDr. R. Poch we aimed at assessing the suitability of the various contrast media used so far. However right from the outset we were aware that the use of any contrast media for obtaining a clearly legible X-ray picture always represents an external disturbance of the natural articulatory process of the speaker.[2]

In the above-mentioned experiments for establishing the most suitable contrast media we radiographed the speech-organs without phonation, with open and closed mouth, during the pronunciation of isolated spoken vowels, and during sung vowels at different pitches. We changed the contrast media (with the same medium we also changed its denseness), and the organs smeared with the medium.

Of the contrast media tested the barium paste came out clearest on the X-ray pictures. Individual parts of the speech-organs were smeared in different combinations with various concentrations of the barium paste to arrive at the desired clarity. So

---

also its height. He introduced the wire through the nasal cavity back to the upper wall of the soft palate. The strength of the closure he established with the aid of hydraulic pressure; lying down he had a small amount of water passed by a tube to the rearmost part of the nasal cavity, and with the vowels *u*, *o*, and *i* the water remained in the nose; with *a* however it began to flow out showing that with *a* the closure is weakest if it cannot take even weak water pressure. But it was precisely this latter experiment which evoked doubt as to whether with *a* the soft palate produces a closure at all."

In 1931, that is five years after the appearance of Hála's publication quoted above, there appears in the work of C. F. Parmenter, S. N. Trevino and C. A. Bevans, "A Technique for Radiographing the Organs of Speech During Articulation", *ZEPh* 1 (1931) 63-84, a description of the method they used for recording the articulatory position during the pronunciation of isolated vowels. For emphasising the contours of the tongue they used a small gold chain which the test subject swallowed. The contour of the soft palate was emphasised either by the insertion of an artificial palate with the chain set in it, or a thin lead strip reaching from the front upper incisors to the uvula was stuck directly on the palate. This lead strip was furthermore fixed to the rear wall of the larynx. Fixation means were employed which were quite demanding on the subject being investigated. Exposure lasted several seconds; it was reduced only with the use of 100 mAs.

2 B. Hála in his *Artikulace českých zvuků v roentgenových obrazech* (skiagramech) from 1926 writes of this: "Scheier, whose experience in this field cannot be adequately valued, altogether rejects the use of any contrast media (probably after the unhappy experiences with Schleich's paste which he mixed with nitrate of bismuth – skin cream); if he states that all artificial means applied in the mouth prevent proper articulation, he is right only in so far as concerns Barth's and Meyer's chains." (p. 7).

J. Chlumský in his work *Radiografie francouzských samohlásek a polosamohlásek*, of the year 1938 writes "In order to make the reading of radiographs easier and safer Polland used bismuth carbonate (bismutum carbonicum) and drew with a brush a guide line along the central line of the lips, the tongue and the arch of the oral cavity. By this means of course a foreign body enters the mouth but in such a small quantity that it in no wise hampers articulation, as both our Parisians agreed in admitting. Bismuth is also ideal for the purpose as it is not unpleasant and causes no irritation; in medicine it is a wellknown means and quite harmless." (p. 4).

for example one palatal arch was smeared, or in addition to a slight clarification of the profile, the hard palate, the soft palate, the front and rear of the uvula, and the back wall of the throat were also smeared. In another case the study subject gargled with a diluted barium paste. However in the analyses of the X-ray pictures it was seen that by gargling, the contrast medium covers the whole uvula and the palatal arches with an insufficiently thick layer, which we envisaged, but it was so even that there are no significant contrasts on the photographs. Barium paste applied before the experiment in a very fine streak on the centre line of the tongue rapidly spread in an irregular layer over almost the whole of the oral cavity. When barium solution was sprayed through the lower nasal passage it was shown that a dilute solution flows too quickly over the uvula into the rear part of the oral cavity and does not adhere well to the smooth surface of the mucous membrane.[3]

We consider the use of barium paste as a contrast medium in phonetic work as unsuitable because the barium paste must always stick in a specific – sometimes quite thick – layer on the articulatory organ smeared with it. Moreover the barium paste may become imprinted on various parts of the oral cavity where this is not desirable. On the other hand however, the dampness of the mucous membrane restricts the adhesion of the barium paste where it is most needed. The greatest barrier to the use of barium paste as a contrast medium is the fact that owing to its property of sticking to the smeared organ it may lead for example to blocking of the velopharyngeal passage, which has in turn been a cause of imprecise evaluation of the mutual position of the soft palate and the back wall of the throat during articulation. Therefore when spraying barium solution through the lower nasal passage we could not use a thick solution as this would block the gap between the back wall of the throat and the soft palate so that not even the pressure of the soft palate during an actual velopharyngeal closure could expel the heavy barium paste collected there (v. fig. 1. in the appendix).

In addition to various kinds of barium paste we used other contrast media for spraying the nasopharynx, for example an injection contrast fluid of iodine water soluble preparation (Diodon Spofa). Not even these contrast media however gave satisfactory results for our work.[4]

[3] We have already drawn attention to this in the article J. Ondráčková – R. Poch, "Zur Methodik der Untersuchung der Vokalartikulation beim Gesang". On the possibility of falsifying the true relationship in the velopharyngeal area with the use of contrast media mention is made two years later by L. Croatto and C. Croatto-Martinolli in the article quoted.

When speaking of the requirement of preserving the conditions for natural articulation it is necessary to take into account also the psychical effect on the test subject with the use of any contrast media.

[4] When we obtained the initial pictures we used contrast media as follows: In 12 cases the lips, tongue and uvula were smeared, in 4 cases the uvula was smeared in combination with a spray into the nasal cavity, in 19 cases there was only the spray into the nasal cavity, in 20 cases just the uvula was smeared, in 4 cases a central line was marked and the palatal arch was smeared, in another 4 cases the central line was smeared and the nasal cavity sprayed, in 22 cases the soft palate and the uvula were smeared, in three cases the palatal arches, in one case the soft palate, in one case the

Nor did we consider suitable the use of those new preparations used in bronchography, where the contrast material is bound on carboxymetylcellulose and which forms a film on the bronchial mucous membrane. We eliminated these from our work as their application requires local anaesthesia which would have a strong side-effect on the physiological functioning of the speech-organs.

Departing from the conviction that the best way of research into the articulatory relations in the supraglottal cavities is photography without any impediment to the natural articulation of the test subject, we discovered, worked out, and in practice evaluated the application of a method new to phonetic research work, using the fact that in the oral and nasopharyngeal cavities there is a perfectly natural negative contrast medium i.e. AIR. This natural contrast medium permits of the taking of X-ray pictures with fully satisfactory contours of the articulatory organs both in static pictures and those obtained by serial roentgenography and cineradiography.[5]

In all further studies our X-ray pictures were taken without recourse to any artificial contrast medium. Individual exposures for the individual test subjects were always placed in the hands of a roentgenologist.

2. COMPLEX RECORDING METHOD

It has not been usual during photography of the articulatory action of the speech-organs in phonation to make a parallel sound record.

As mentioned above, we were convinced that the moment of exposure of the photograph will not always catch the sound at its "proper articulation phase". Not even with the test subjects who were professional singers, was it possible in each individual case to establish by ear with the necessary degree of accuracy whether the character of the sound was maintained throughout the whole exposure time, and at what intensity and pitch it was realised. This was not even possible after preliminary tests were carried out. For these reasons we considered it essential to make up a reproduceable sound record of the sound simultaneously with the exposure of the picture. It was an additional essential requirement that a precise indication be made of what part of the articulation is recorded on the X-ray picture for the duration of the exposure. To this end we elaborated and tested a complex recording method, i.e. a method of synchronised sound and oscillograph recording which precisely corresponded to the exposure time of the X-ray picture.

First of all it was necessary to try to find the best lighting and film speed for copying

nasopharynx was emphasised, in three cases the test subject gargled with the contrast medium and then swallowed it, in 48 cases the central line was marked with contrast medium, in 48 cases only the lips, in 78 cases the lips in combination with a light smearing of the tip of the tongue.

5 166 static pictures were obtained without the use of any contrast medium as were also all the serial roentgenograms and the three parts of the cineradiographic film.

the curves from the oscilloscope screen with a camera with continuous film transport.[6] When we used the ordinary screen the film was underexposed at relatively slow film speeds. This failing was overcome by the use of an oscilloscope with a cathode-ray tube with acceleration voltage and with a blue trace which we used in all our later experiments.[7]

For the synchronous records we had necessarily to construct an automatic switch. (fig. 1.)

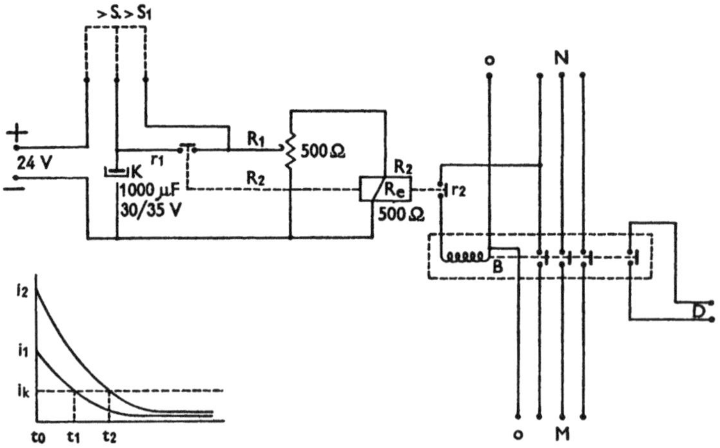

Fig. 1. Plan of the automatic switch. S,S1 – automatic switch, K – condenser, Re – relay, B – electromagnetic switch, N – lead, D – Bucky screen switch, M – film camera motor.

The automatic switch is constructed so that pressure on the button links up the operation of the oscillograph, the film camera for copying the curves and the power supply of the rotating-anode of the X-ray tube. The switch automatically exposed the X-ray picture with a delay of 0.2 sec. which corresponded to the full run of the rotating-anode used in the X-ray apparatus. During the exposure of the X-ray picture a light signal is automatically activated on the oscilloscope screen, so that the section of the oscilloscope curve filmed by the camera and accurately corresponding to the exposure time of the X-ray picture, is marked by the light signal check.[8]

The source of the light signal is a small bulb located at the lower edge of the oscilloscope screen. The bulb with low inertia produced in the rhythm of the network frequency a broken light-line on the lower edge of the film record of the oscilloscope curve. (fig. 2.)

With the complex recording method we took static roentgenograms in the following time sequence: after the tape-recorder, the oscillograph and the X-ray ap-

[6] The first experiment was carried out in April 1956.

[7] We filmed with a Meopta camera adapted for the higher speed of the continuous film transport at 5 m/s on TF 4 film. The sound recording was made on Pyral tape at a rate of 16.2 cm/s.

[8] The automatic switch was constructed by Ing. V. Palička and Ing. V. Maláč.

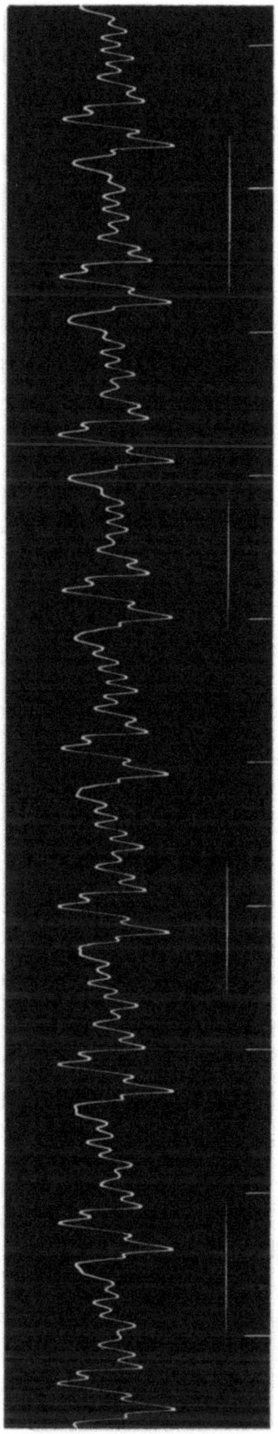

Fig. 2. Oscilloscopic record with a light indication of the exposure of X-ray film. The trace of light at the bottom edge appears in the rhythm of the circuit frequency.

paratus were brought into action the test subject began to phonate the relevant vowel. At the appropriate moment (usually after a trial run) the button of the automatic switch brought simultaneously into motion the camera for photographing the oscilloscopic curve, and the rotating-anode of the X-ray tube. 0.2 second later the switch automatically exposed an X-ray picture and for the duration of the exposure switched in automatically the interrupted light signal on the oscilloscope screen. By releasing the button the switch ceased to function when the sound of the rotating anode was independently registered on the sound record.

The test subject sat in a separate room linked to the X-ray inspection room by a narrow door which was partially compacted with felt wadding. The tape-recorder, the oscilloscope and the camera were in another insulated room. In this way we managed to prevent the sound of the camera penetrating to the tape-recorder and the noise from the rotating-anode of the X-ray tube was considerably damped. (fig. 3.)

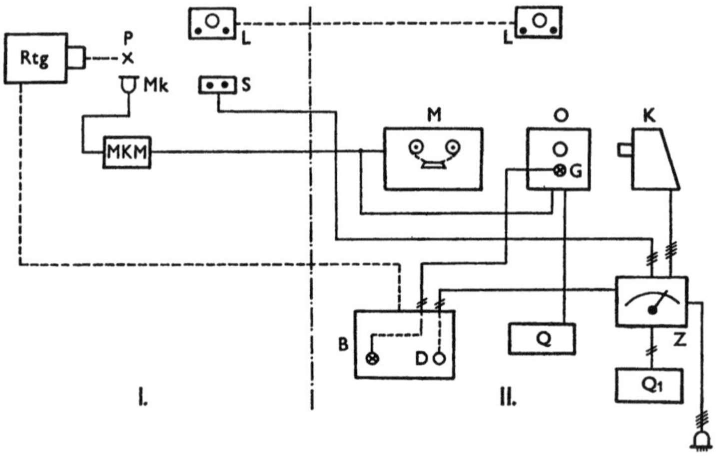

Fig. 3. Diagram showing the apparatus linked up for the complex method. I. Work room: Rtg – X-ray apparatus, P – test subject, Mk – microphone, MKM – microphone amplifier, S – electromagnetic automatic switch. II. Ancillary room: M – tape-recorder, O – oscillograph, G – bulb for the light recording during the exposition of the film, K – film camera, Z – electromagnetic time switch, D – Bucky screen, B – control desk of the X-ray apparatus, Q,Q_1 – sources of tension, L – communication mechanism which connects both rooms.

By the above-mentioned ordering of events we obtained a sound record and a photograph of the oscilloscope curve of the phonation of the vowel before the switching on of the rotating-anode of the X-ray tube, a sound record and a photograph of the oscilloscope curve during phonation of the vowel through the exposure time of the X-ray shot, and a sound record and photograph of the realisation of the vowel with the simultaneous noise of the X-ray tube after the exposure of the photograph, and finally a record of only the noise of the rotating-anode of the X-ray tube. (figs. 4a, b, c)

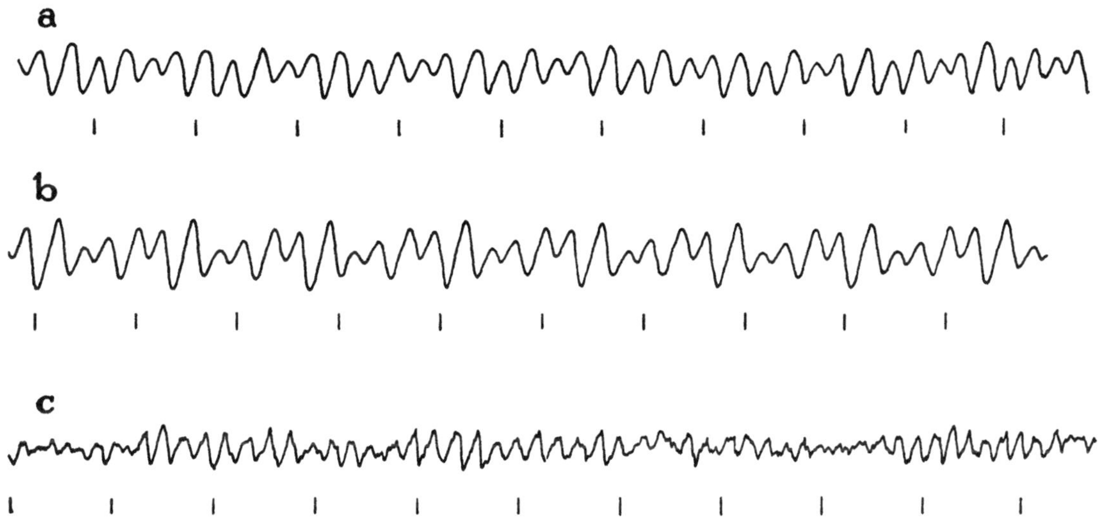

Fig. 4. Oscilloscopic records (a) of the vowel *ó* without the noise of the X-ray tube (5 *ó* 110 dB), (b) of the vowel *ó* with the noise of the X-ray tube (7 *ó* + rsg 110 dB), (c) of the noise of the X-ray tube (6 rsg 85 dB).

The recording of the noise of the X-ray apparatus also depended on the spatial location of the microphone (quite significant can be the role of stationary waves and reflection).[9]

The use of this method of complex recording since 1956 has afforded us the following advantages:

1. It fixes accurately what phase of the articulation of the vowel is registered on the X-ray picture, and tells us what is its acoustic character.

2. The tape record represented the whole phonation and included the noise made by switching on and off the camera with the automatic switch. Before the operation of the X-ray apparatus the realisation of the vowel without the noise of the rotating-anode of the X-ray tube was recorded on the tape, and after phonation there was the plain record of the noise of the X-ray tube alone.

[9] For the sound recording we used a Philips tape-recorder and a condensor microphone VÚT which was placed 10cm from the mouth of the test subject. The optical record was made on a Philips GM 5256 (oscilloscope screen with a blue spot, accelerating anode DB 9-5, accelerating voltage 3kV); the trace was filmed with a Meopta KP 1 camera.

We did not succeed in eliminating altogether the disturbing noise of the rotating-anode of the X-ray tube, because in our provisional work-place it was impossible always to carry out all the necessary sound insulation without interrupting the daily work of the X-ray section of the clinic. The use of a portable sound-insulated cabin provoked a feeling of awkwardness in the test subject and coloured his subjective hearing of his own voice.

A throat microphone which would have eliminated the disturbing noise of the X-ray tube was not suitable because it registered sound in a perverted form. Even the test subject felt it as an unnatural interference. A gradient microphone was also unsuitable for our purposes owing to its inadequate frequency range.

3. We could always at any time later check the acoustic quality of the vowel against the sound recording and carry out an analysis of it.

4. All the above-mentioned synchronous records gave us material which can at any time later be subjected to investigation under conditions as close as possible to those at the time of the original realisation.

As supplementary method we studied the nostril sound.

The study of whether the nasal cavity is included in or excluded from direct participation in articulation is rendered difficult by the fact that the resonance of the nasal cavity is operative even when there is a complete velopharyngeal closure. This is proved by the fact that even during the articulation of vowels with a firm velopharyngeal closure a microphone placed by the nostrils registers wavy motions which can be observed on the oscillograph.[10] We obtain a similar oscilloscope curve if we place a microphone to the parietal bone of a test subject during phonation.

The velopharyngeal passage during phonation can only show then a direct air current entering into the nasal cavity. We tried to record this air current directly by microphone without the introduction of a nozzle. The oral current was led off by a tube fitted with a proper mouthpiece. Then we tried to record only the oral current and led off the nasal current with a nostril hose. One might however expect that with the use of any such hose there would be such deformation that the records would lose all practical significance.[11]

We achieved the best results when we registered with a double-beam oscillograph and condenser microphone the nasal current by placing the microphone close up to the nostrils leaving only a narrow passage, and at the same time with another micro-

[10] For the measurement of acoustic pressure in the nasal and oral cavities we obtained a special sounding device in cooperation with Tesla. The pressure of the oral and nasal air currents has been investigated for example by H. Krech. With the German vowels whose acoustic form is barely distinct from that of Czech vowels in his observations, he did not find a firm velopharyngeal closure in the majority of cases. ("Über ein einfaches Verfahren zur Aufzeichnung des oralen und nasalen Schalldruckanteiles gesprochner Sprache, Aktuelle Probleme der Phoniatrie und Logopädie", Supplement *FPh* 1 [1960] 100-108.)

In this connection H. H. Wängler writes: "Das Gaumensegel gibt im Deutschen nur bei den Nasalen /*m*, *n*, *ŋ*/ den Nasenweg ganz frei, während es ihn bei allen anderen Lauten mehr oder weniger behindert bzw. versperrt. Bekannt war, dass nicht etwa das Zäpfchen diese Arbeit verrichtet /das hängt stets herunter/, sondern das Velum durch Hebung die Annäherung an den Passavantschen Wulst besorgt. Neu ist m. W. die an den vorliegenden Ergebnissen gemachte Beobachtung, dass es lautgerechte Grade der Annäherung gibt, die offensichtlich einem bestimmten Gesetz folgen. Sie scheinen nämlich durchaus von der oralen Engebildung abhängig zu sein. Ist der Mundweg vollkommen frei /z.B. bei *a*/, so ist die Abschliessungstendenz am geringsten, wird er jedoch auf verschiedene Weise mehr und mehr verlegt /*ε* – *e* – *i* oder *o* – *u* – *y*/, so wächst sie, bis sie über die Reibelaute mit den Verschlusslauten am grössten wird. Jetzt wird völlige Absperrung des Nasenweges tatsächlich erreicht. Das Gaumensegel richtet sich damit hinsichtlich seiner Funktion bei der Lautgebung nach der jeweils gegebenen artikulatorischen Notwendigkeit." (*Atlas deutscher Sprachtaute*, Berlin, 1961, p. 19 n.).

[11] A review of the works concerned with the investigation of air pressure (acoustic pressure), or tension of the articulatory organs, is given by E. Fischer-Jørgensen and A. T. Hansen in the article "An Electrical Manometer and its Use in Phonetic Research", *Phonetica* 4 (1959) 43-53.

phone recording simultaneously the oral and nasal currents. This second microphone was placed about 40 cm from the mouth.

In subsequent experiments it is necessary always to bear in mind that the size of the nasal cavity during phonation is practically constant, whereas the size of the oral cavity changes considerably with the movement of the tongue and the soft palate and by the change in the jaw angle, as has been mentioned above.

3. SKETCHES

From the X-ray pictures we took sketches of the mobile parts of the speech-organs for normal study purposes.

We made widest use in obtaining the sketches from the X-ray pictures of drawings of the outline contours of the speech organs on translucent paper.[12] The sketches can then be reproduced in a variety of ways. Some authors trace the contours of the soft parts of the speech-organs directly from the original X-ray pictures and then reproduce the latter.[13] In this way however the original X-ray picture is damaged.

A sketch affords a very clear, in some cases a schematic, picture of the articulation phase of the speech-organs during the realisation of the given sound. And in spite of every effort taken to ensure an objective record the sketch nevertheless contains signs of individual interpretation, so that not even a very finely drawn curve expresses as a rule the fineness of the contour of the articulatory organs being studied.

In order to preserve the original X-ray pictures which are with the application of the newly elaborated method of complex recording an inseparable and very important part of the material obtained as a whole, we took by photographic means good quality copies of the X-ray originals for our further work. After many experiments and technical tests we also obtained positive copies of the X-ray pictures on which all the necessary details were as clearly visible as on the originals.

A detailed study requires of course detailed analyses of a large number of X-ray pictures from different points of view.

X-ray photographs were analysed in such a way that we studied them closely on X-ray illuminator, described the phases of movement of the articulatory organs during phonation of the given vowel after the principles reading of X-ray pictures in roentgenologic practice, drew a sketch (or schematic diagram), and prepared a good-quality photocopy of the roentgenogram. With this treatment the evaluation of X-ray films is made to a great degree objective by comparison with the interpretation of

[12] This method is normal at the Prague phonetics school. Viz for example the continuously changed and improved development of sketches in B. Hála, K. Ohnesorg, M. Romportl, A. Skaličková.
[13] E.g. R. Husson; B. Hála made sketches by emphasising the contours of the speech-organs directly on the positive copies of the roentgenograms when he then treated chemically such that only the drawing remained. (B. Polland – B. Hála, op. cit.)

them by means of sketches without preservation of the originals. Many methods have been worked out for the reading of roentgenograms by different authors.[14]

During our analyses of the roentgenograms we first made observations of the lip formations, then those of the tongue and the soft palate during the realisation of the vowel, then the consequences of all this for the size of the mouth and throat cavities; for sung vowels pitch and tonal intensity was always registered.

4. EXPOSURE OF THE X-RAY FILMS

It is also necessary to devote great attention to the most suitable time of exposure, and to other technical parameters in the obtaining of X-ray films. These parameters are always settled by a roentgenologist, and moreover separately for each test subject.

5. OBJECTIVE MEASURING OF THE X-RAY PHOTOGRAPHS

To a considerable degree subjective elements in the evaluation of X-ray pictures have been eliminated for us by the use of the method of objective measuring of them. It depends on the fact that for reading off the important parameters on the X-ray pictures for phonetic purposes we use appropriate photoresistors,[15] whose sensitivity

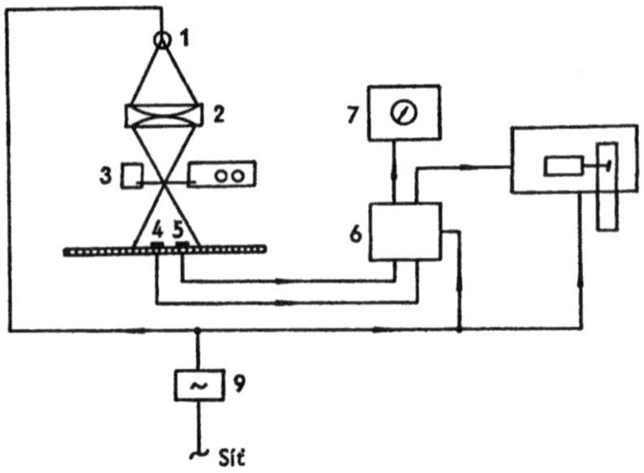

Fig. 5. Block diagram of the apparatus used in the objective analysis of roentgenograms. 1. light source, 2. condenser, 3. X-ray pictures (film), 4 and 5 appropriate photoresistors, 6. differential transformer of the DC – AC signal, 7. voltmeter, 8. electromechanic recorder, 9. stabiliser of the circuit tension. (Diagram after Ing. S. Hlaváč.)

[14] For some details see for example J. W. Tuddenham, The Visual Physiology of Roentgen Diagnosis, *AJR* 78 (1957) 116-123. We also tried out his method of using lenses for the reading of roentgenograms. A reducing lense increases the gradient of light contrasts so much that it makes the study of the picture easier.

[15] Viz J. Aulich, "Fotoelektrické odpory spékané s přívodními elektrodami", *SO* 22 (1961) 397-401; J. Ondráčková, "Objektivní analýzy rentgenogramů mluvidel", *ČSAV* Věstník 71 (1962) 558-559.

to changes in lighting is suitably adapted for light contrasts in the X-ray picture, and so enable us to register objectively these changes. Because we make no use of any contrast media in our X-ray photography, no layer of contrast medium nor any other change in lightness which might be caused by dispersed contrast medium appears on the X-ray picture.

The parameters which mark the contours of the soft parts of the speech-organs are evaluated against the graphic record obtained from the Brüel and Kjaer recorder.[16] They can also be read off on the scale of a measuring apparatus (voltmeter, ohmmeter). (fig. 5.)

The application of photoresistors in the analysis of cineradiographic shots requires particularly special technical solution.

6. THE METHOD OF COMPARATIVE ANALYSIS: THE ANALYSIS OF CINERADIOGRAPHIC SHOTS WITH THE AID OF FILM LOOPS

The method of comparative analysis enables us to observe the movements of the speech-organs with a sound accompaniment during the phonation of vowels, syllables

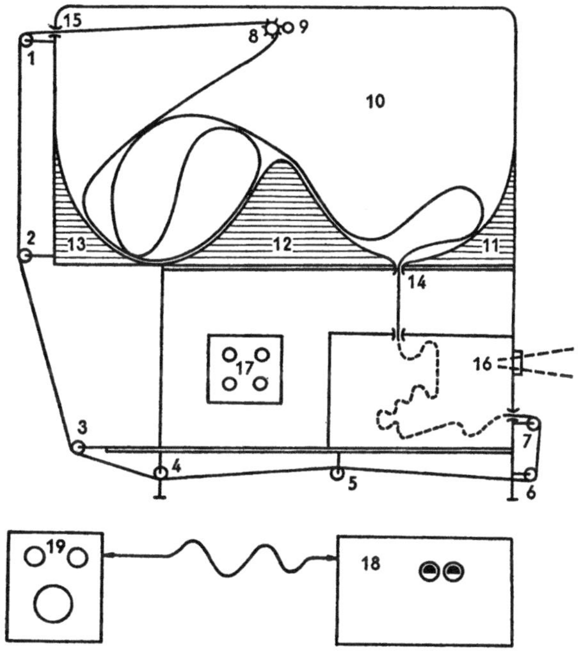

Fig. 6. Diagram of the movement of the film loop in the adaptor. 1-7 mobile pulleys carrying the film loop, 8. driving pulley, 9. adhering pulley, 10. space for film loop, 11-13. space freed to let the film loop glide more easily, 14-15. smoothed off passages, 16. 35 mm sound projector, 17. switch control board, 18. sound amplifier, 19. reproducers. (Diagram after Ing. Hlaváč.)

[16] The construction of the apparatus was worked out in cooperation with Ing. S. Hlaváč.

and greater units. It is of particular value to the phonetician in that in the evaluation of the results of the analysis we can turn our attention to the various correlations of the individual phonetic phenomena. A further advantage of this method is that we are aware of and analyse just those most marked and most characteristic features which are relevant or which seem to be relevant to the movement of the speech-organs over the whole period of articulation of the given vowel.

The comparative analysis of the cineradiographic shots of the movement of the speech-organs during phonation is carried out in the following way. We project the film loops of varying length from an adapted sound projector (35 mm) taken from the copy of the cineradiographic film. These allows us to reproduce in unbroken sequence the sound and picture of the speech-organs in motion during phonation.[17] (fig. 6.)

The use of loops proved to be very sound because: (a) there is no need to interrupt the projection – the eye remains well accommodated to the reading of the X-ray shots; (b) during several repetitions of the projection the characteristic features of the action of the speech-organs are more clearly expressed; and (c) it allows the observation of the natural course of the movement of the speech-organs in a repeated realisation with an assurance of there being the same conditions.

[17] The adaptor was produced in the Phonetics Laboratory of ČSAV, Praha.

III

ANALYSES OF THE ARTICULATORY PROCESS ON THE BASIS OF PLANE FILMS AND SERIAL ROENTGENOGRAMS

The articulatory position of the speech-organs during the realisation of spoken Czech long vowels was described as early as 1926 by B. Hála on the basis of static X-ray pictures (skiagrams).[1] The activity of the speech-organs during sung and whispered Czech vowels[2] is now being analysed for the first time. During sung vowels there is a greater degree of change in pitch and tone intensity, and their mutual combination. There is the added influence of various types of voice training and professional singing practice. A full-scale investigation of these questions requires still more painstaking research, as it must be understood in all its complexity.

In analyses of the photographs obtained by the methods which show the articulatory phase of the phonation of vowels, we concentrated on the articulatory organs in the supraglottal cavities. By their mobility and combinations of their relative positions they shape and modify the size of the mouth and throat cavities and the passage to the nasal cavity.[3] These modifications act together in the production of certain very significant specific acoustic qualities of the vowels, by which the individual vowels are distinguished.

For detailed analyses we took 433 static plane X-ray films including roentgenograms obtained by the modified stereoscopic method. For this purpose we had the cooperation of 16 test subjects (6 women and 10 men). For the final analyses we used

1 B. Polland – B. Hála, *Artikulace českých zvuků v roentgenových obrazech* (skiagramech), Praha 1926.

2 More recently work has been carried out on phonation in singing for example by R. Husson (v. bibliography) and the workers of the acoustics laboratory at the Moscow Conservatory. Among the Czech authors K. Sedláček has been most occupied with this problem (Akustická analýza zpěvního hlasu", *ČLČ* 101, 1962, pp. 291-296). The musical factors of speech and the question of the physiology of hearing the melody of speech are taken up by K. Sedláček – A. Sychra in the publication *Hudba a slovo z experimentálního hlediska*, Praha 1962.

3 The designations of the individual supraglottal cavities do not overlap terminologically in anatomy and phonetics. So for example in phonetics the oral cavity reaches the rear wall of the throat (pharynx) while in medicine the distinction is made between the oral cavity and the oropharynx; the nasal cavity in the phonetic sense is divided from the medical point of view into nasal cavity and nasopharynx. The throat cavity according to phonetic terminology borders on the oral cavity and reaches as far as the larynx. Where according to the anatomical division the oral cavity ends, the glottal cavity begins, and this is divided into nasopharynx and oropharynx (after B. Hála – M. Sovák, *Hlas – řeč – sluch*, Praha 1962 4, p. 97, from where is also taken the schematic representation in figs. 7a, b).

the evaluations of the photographs of three men and two women, i.e. 256 shots. Of these 119 were of articulation during sung vowels, 70 during spoken vowels, 50 during whispered vowels, 6 during a neutral nasal sound and 11 roentgenograms showing the speech-organs without phonation. The remaining shots, particularly the trials and the initial ones which were obtained while we were still looking for new methods were not included in the final evaluation. Detailed notes were taken as the work progressed.[4]

The analyses were classified according to the individual vowels in the order *í*, *é*, *á*, *ó*, *ú*, first the sung vowels only, then the spoken and whispered ones. Finally for the sake of comparison we carried out analyses of the speech organs during a neutral nasal sound, and without phonation with closed and open mouth.[5]

Pitch was established with a tuning fork; intensity of the tone was changed on the normal relative degrees of piano, mezzoforte and forte.

Insofar as we give any concrete measures in millimeters in our analyses, taken from the roentgenograms, they do not represent actual size; however they are all on the

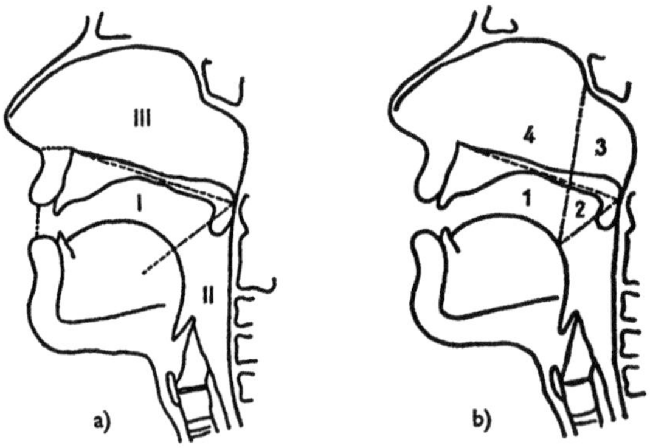

Fig. 7. Schematic representation of the designation of the supraglottal cavities (a) according to phonetic terminology: I – oral cavity, II – throat cavity, III – nasal cavity; (b) according to medical terminology: 1 – oral cavity, 2 – oropharynx, 3 – nasopharynx, 4 – nasal cavity. (After B. Hála – M. Sovák, *Hlas – řeč – sluch*, Praha 1951).

4 In the notes made at the time of the experiments are recorded the date of the radiographing, the place, the name of the test subject, his vocal register, the vowel to be realised (pitch and intensity), information as to whether it is to be sung, spoken or whispered, whether it is to be a neutral sound or the speech-organs are without phonation, with the mouth open or closed, also kind of X-ray film, the type of X-ray apparatus, the number of the shot, the exposure time, the method of development, and the X-ray method employed; from the beginning was also recorded the kind of contrast medium and information as to which parts of the articulatory organs were smeared with the contrast medium, and how this was done.

5 Numerals on the sketches indicate the order number of the original roentgenogram according to the basic report and is the same as the number of the copy and the sketch.

For example information about the analysed roentgenogram RJ 322-323 – Z í (a^1) mf s, means that it is a matter of the analysis of the sung vowel *í* at pitch a^1 and intensity mezzoforte; it was realised by test subject RJ, and pictures 322-323 were obtained by the modified stereoscopic /s/ method. Z = sung; M = spoken; Š = whispered.

same scale in the case of shots obtained by the same method (from roentgenograms somewhat increased, on copies – reproductions – reduced).

The significance of serial roentgenograms for phonetic research in articulation is in no wise reduced by the fact that it is now possible to record the movements of the speech-organs during phonation by the cineradiographic method. On the contrary the use of a combination of both methods (possibly even with other methods, e.g. tomographic or stereoscopic) will always be very useful as these methods complement each other particularly well.

By the method of serial roentgenography we obtained in all 757 shots, of which for our work we took 460.[6]

Unlike the case of the static roentgenograms compared according to the individual vowels in the realisation of the various test subjects, it was necessary in the analysis of the serial roentgenograms to maintain in the reproduction of the shots the order of the individual phases of phonation recorded on the continuous strip of X-ray film of the serial roentgenogram. Because the method of serial roentgenography allows of a minimal rate of four shots per second, it could be used for recording the separate partial phases of articulation during the phonation of the natural unit of articulation – the long syllable.[7]

One should be aware that film speed is, relative to its width, very fast (with 30 × 30 cm pictures at 4 exposures a second the film is shifting at 4 × 30 cm per second).

As has already been mentioned this method is very suitable for the observation of the details of articulation, (serial roentgenograms give a somewhat enlarged image of the speech organs).

1. THE SPEECH-ORGANS DURING THE ARTICULATION OF THE VOWEL *í*

From the analayses of the roentgenograms recording the formation of the speech-organs during the articulation of spoken, sung and whispered *í* (or *í* in the syllable *bí*) some conclusions which we here place alongside the already published descriptions of the articulation of vowels in Czech.[8] (figs. 8, 9, 10, 11.)

[6] At the request of the Theatre Institute of the Ministry of Education 300 shots were taken recording the articulation of the speech organs during singing of a continuous extract of a song. This was done for the sake of the cooperative resolution of certain specific problems.

[7] Here we are concerned with registering the entirely natural articulation of a spoken syllable with a long vowel or a long sung syllable, and the transition phenomena which are lacking for instance by Kirkpatrick in the cineradiographic films acquired so far. (J. A. Kirkpatrick – R. W. Olmsted, "Cinefluorographic Study of Pharyngeal Function Related to Speech", *Radiology* 73 [1959] 557-559.) These requirements are for the purposes of phonetics fulfilled to a large extent by serial roentgenography and even more by cineradiography. The requirement of a synchronnous sound recording was supplied in our material in 1957 by the introduction of the complex method.

[8] For example B. Hála, *Fonetické obrazy hlásek*, Praha 1960; *Uvedení do fonetiky češtinyr na obecně fonetickém základě*, Praha 1962.

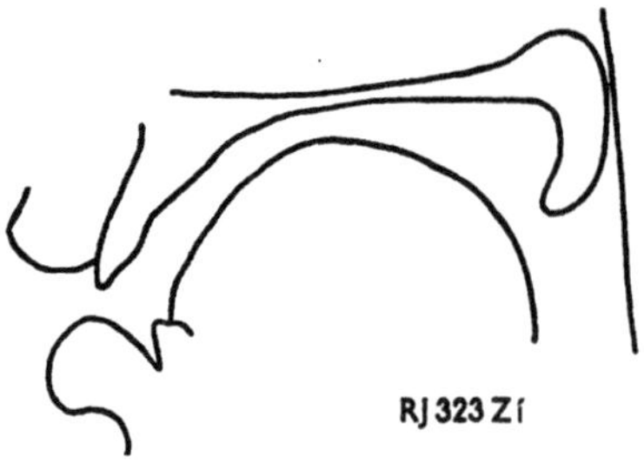

Fig. 8. Sung *i* (a^1) mf, RJ 323, s. The lips are 10 mm apart. The tongue is almost regularly arched forwards and upwards and in its middle section the crest approaches the hard palate at a distance of 6 mm. The tip of the tongue lies against the lower incisors. The soft palate is fairly strongly tonized (it is above the level of the hard palate), but it does not touch the rear wall of the throat, so that a narrow passage is left to the nasal cavity. The uvula points with its tip toward the oral cavity. The width of the throat cavity (20 mm) is characteristic for the vowel *i*.

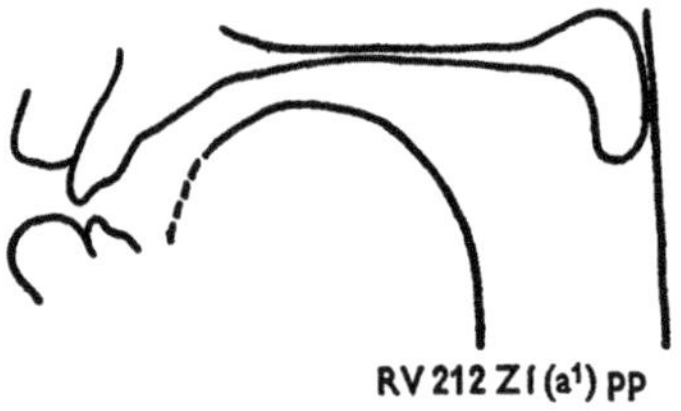

Fig. 9. Sung *i* (a^1) pp, RV 212, s. The lips are held open at a distance of 8 mm apart. The tongue is strongly tonized. The summit of its arch is 7 mm from the hard palate. The soft palate is also strongly tonized but the passage to the nasal cavity remains open; in the area of the rear face of the uvula there is a hairbreadth gap which widens upwards first to 1 mm then higher to 2 mm. The width of the throat cavity reaches 30 mm.

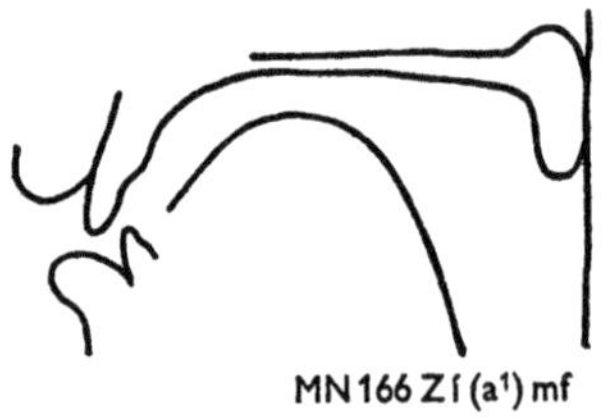

Fig. 10. Sung *i* (a^1) mf, MN 166, s. The distance between the lips measures 7 mm. The tongue is arched forwards and upwards towards the hard palate, from which its summit is 5 mm distant. The throat cavity reaches a width of 23 mm in the area of the root of the tongue. The soft palate has marked tonus and the passage to the nasal cavity is firmly closed.

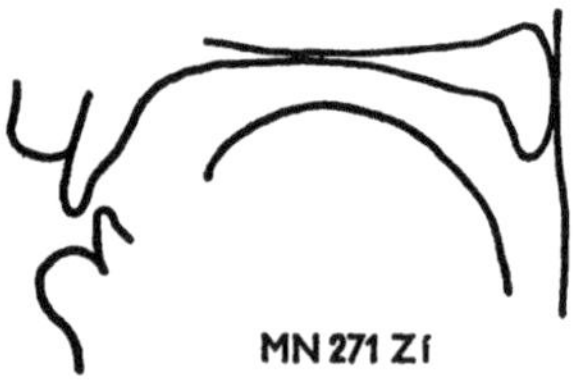

Fig. 11. Sung *i* (e^2) mf, MN 271, s. The distance between the lips is 16 mm. The tip of the tongue points towards the lower incisors. The back of the tongue is arched upwards and forwards and approaches the hard palate to a distance of 8 mm. The soft palate firmly closes the passage to the nasal cavity. The throat cavity is particularly narrow (7 mm).

During sung *i* the capacity of the front part of the oral cavity is characteristically larger then with spoken *i*, but even during sung *i* it is small by comparison with the other vowels. The crest of the tongue follows the alveolae and the hard palate at a regular distance. It is regularly arched with the summit of the crest considerably closer to the hard palate. The tongue is thrust forwards and upwards, so that it considerably liberates the space in the throat cavity, which is at its largest with the vowel *i* by comparison with the other vowels. The tip of the tongue touches the back of the lower incisors.[9] (figs. 12, 13, 14, 15.)

[9] Only in two cases did the tip of the tongue not rest against the lower incisors: sketch MN 271

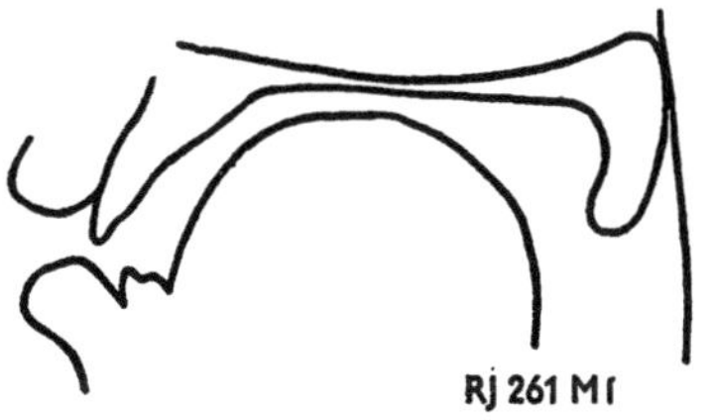

Fig. 12. Spoken *í* RJ 261, s. The lips are 7 mm apart. The tongue is arched. It follows the arch of the hard palate at a distance of 3-4 mm. The soft palate is raised. Its upper contour forms an arch. In its upper third the rear wall of the soft palate lightly touches the rear wall of the throat and closes the passage to the nasal cavity.

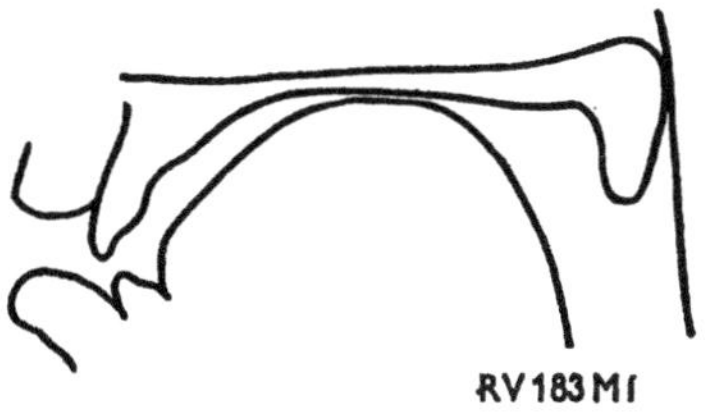

Fig. 13. Spoken *í* RV 183, s. The lips are 8 mm apart. The tip of the tongue is behind the lower incisors. Its crest is abruptly arched almost touching the hard palate, and in its rear part it drops away downwards. The soft palate has strong tonus and is raised upwards and backwards. On picture 182 there is a millimeter-wide passage to the nasal cavity, while on 183 the passage to the nasal cavity is firmly closed. The width of the throat cavity measures 20 mm.

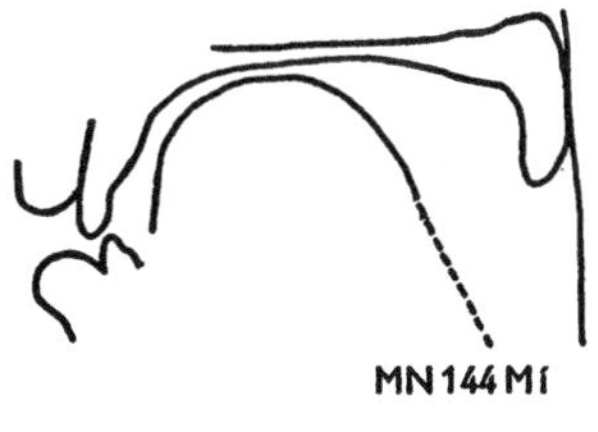

Fig. 14. Spoken *í* MN 144, s. The distance between the lips is 8 mm. The tongue follows the arch of the hard palate at a distance of 2-3 mm. The summit of the arch of the tongue is thrust forwards and upwards. The soft palate has tonus. Its upper contour is predominantly level. That part of the soft palate by the rear wall of the throat is however thrust up to a higher level by about 2 mm. The velopharyngeal closure is firm. The width of the throat cavity narrows progressively downwards; at the level of the uvula it reaches 25 mm.

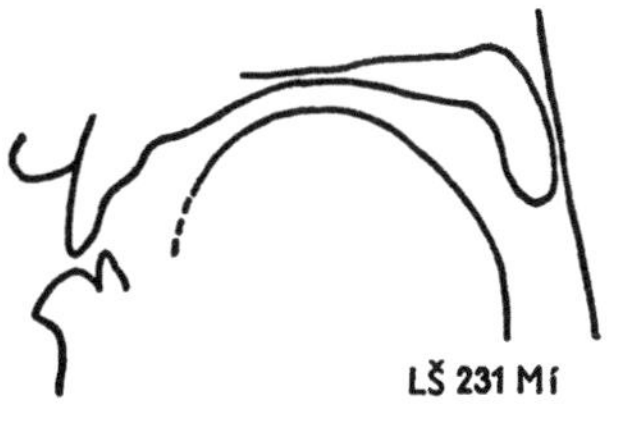

Fig. 15. Spoken *í* LŠ 231, s. The lips are wide apart – 15 mm. The tongue is arched up in the middle part of its crest. From the hard palate it is 3 mm distant. The soft palate has weak tonus. Its upper contour undulates mildly twice. In the area of the uvula it approaches the rear wall of the throat. The passage to the nasal cavity remains open however.

If we look at the measurements we state that the distance of the crest of the tongue from the alveolae and the hard palate is least during whispered *í*, a little greater during spoken *í*, and almost twice the size during sung *í*.[10] The higher the tone, the greater is the distance between the crest of the tongue and the alveolae.[11] (figs. 16, 17, 18, 19.)

Z *í* (e^2) (fig. 11), where there is a markedly clear raising of the tip of the tongue; sketch RV 212 Z *í* (a^1) (fig. 9) where there is also an extraordinarily wide throat cavity.

10 E.g. in RJ during *í* whispered (Š) the shortest distance is 3 mm, during *í* spoken (M) 3-5 mm and during *í* sung (Z) 6 mm; in AM the distance is 2-3 mm during *í* M and 5-8 mm during *í* Z.

11 E.g. sketch 166 (MN *í* Z a^1) and 271 (MN *í* Z e^2) (fig. 10 and 11).

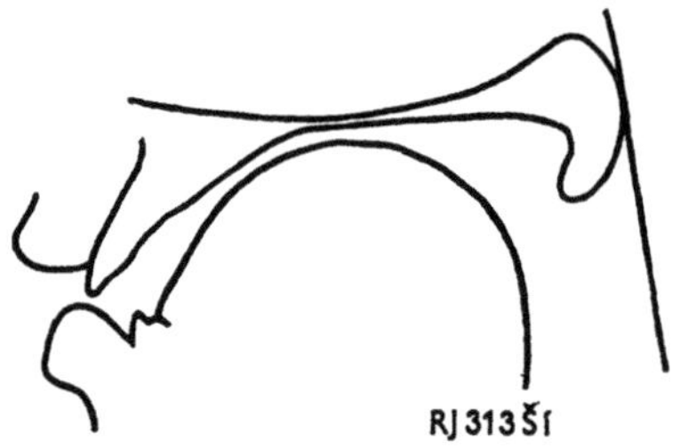

Fig. 16. Whispered *í* RJ 313, s. The distance between the lips measures 6 mm. The tongue is in a smooth drawn out arch directed upwards and forwards to the hard palate which it approaches to a distance of 3 mm. The tip of the tongue is behind the upper edge of the lower incisors. Tonus on the tongue is marked, as is that of the soft palate which closes the passage to the nasal cavity. The width of the throat cavity is 23 mm.

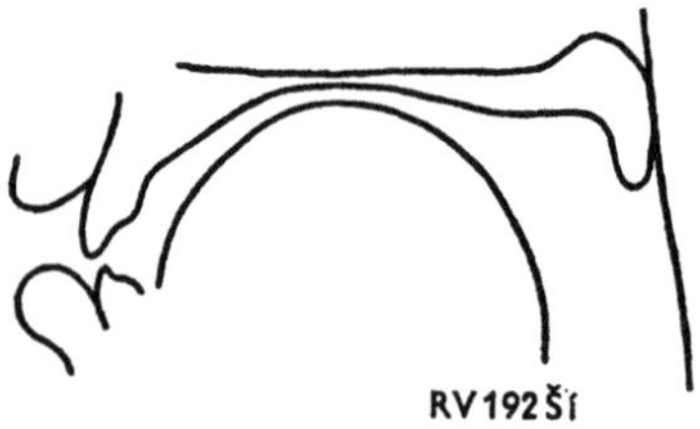

Fig. 17. Whispered *í* RV 192, s. The lips are 9 mm apart. The tongue has strong tonus. In its central section it is arched almost up to the hard palate. The tonus of the soft palate is stronger than with spoken *í*. The passage to the nasal cavity is firmly closed. The width of the throat cavity reaches 20 mm.

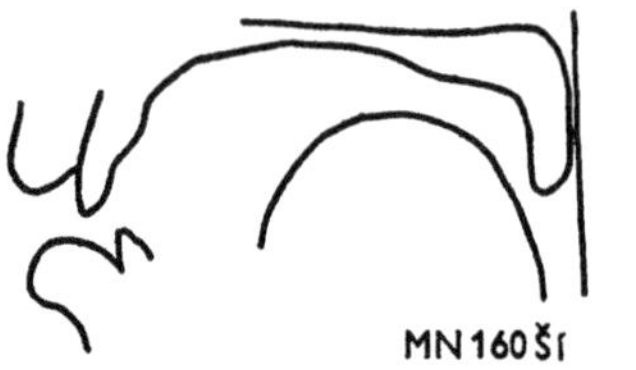

Fig. 18. Whispered *í* MN 160, s. The labial aperture measures 8 mm. The summit of the arch of the tongue is directed towards the soft palate but remains 7 mm away from it. As against spoken *í* the tongue is thrust slightly backwards and upwards so that the throat cavity is relatively narrow (15 mm). The shape of the arching of the tongue corresponds to the shape of the tongue in the same person with sung *í*. The tonus of the soft palate is weak. Between its rear face and the rear wall of the throat there is a gap.

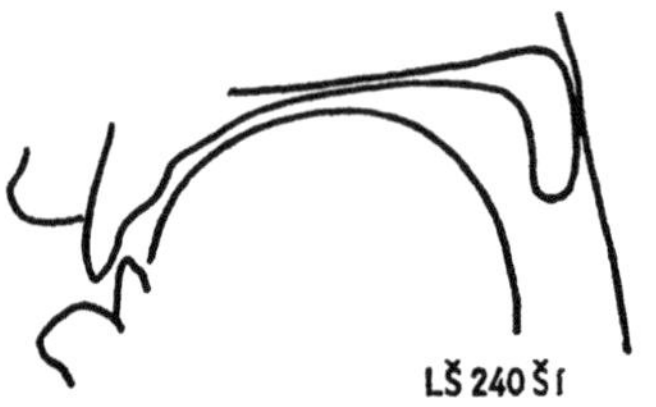

Fig. 19. Whispered *í* LŠ 240, s. The distance between the lips is 14 mm. The arch of the front part of the crest of the tongue follows the alveolae at a distance of 3 mm. The rear section of the crest of the tongue falls away parallel with the rear wall of the throat at a distance of 17 mm. The soft palate has stronger tonus than during spoken *í*. It is in contact with the rear wall of the throat. The width of the throat cavity measures 26 mm.

The width of the gap between the lips does not vary greatly between sung *í* and spoken and whispered *í*. From the measurements we cannot derive any direct dependence of the width between the lips either on the pitch or on the intensity of the tone.[12]

12 Here are some of the values measured: shots HŠ 639-646 Z b*í* (a^1) – labial gap 18 mm, during b*í* M of shots 192-194 the labial gap is 17 mm, on JD 727-731 Z b*í* mf (a^1) it is 12 mm, on 161-164 M b*í* it is again 12 mm. On test subject MN the following measurements were made for the width of the labial gap: shot 166 *í* Z (a^1) – 7 mm, 434 *í* Z (a^1) – 9 mm, 270 *í* Z (e^2) – 16 mm, 144 *í* M – 8 mm, 424 *í* M – 7 mm, 160 *í* Š – 8 mm; on subject LŠ the measurements were: for shot 448 *í* Z – 12 mm, 230 *í* M – 15 mm, 240 *í* Š – 14 mm, etc.

The tonus of the tongue can be marked as strong as the whole tongue is thrust forwards and upwards, by which as we have indicated, the throat cavity is considerably widened.[13] The tonus of the soft palate is in all cases of sung *í* strong to very strong. The velopharyngeal closure is however firmer with spoken *í* than with sung *í*. In some cases, in spite of the very strong tonus of the soft palate and the uvula, the passage to the nasal cavity remains open. A very tight closure is accompanied by a marked arching of the upper contour of the soft palate in an upward direction and by a pressing of its rear wall against the rear wall of the throat which actively contributes to the contact. The velopharyngeal closure in these cases reaches a considerable length.[14]

2. THE SPEECH-ORGANS DURING THE ARTICULATION OF THE VOWEL *é*

The articulatory formation of the speech-organs during phonation of the sung vowel *é* is distinct from their formation during the phonation of spoken *é*. Whereas the oral cavity is only slightly larger during spoken *é* then during sung, spoken and whispered *í*, during sung *é* it is considerably larger.[15] (figs. 20, 21, 22.)

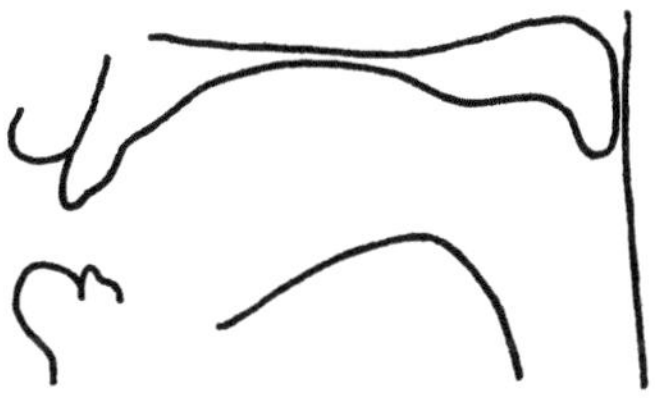

Fig. 20. Sung *é* (a^1) pp, RV 215, s. The lips are 14 mm apart. The tonus of the tongue is mild as is that of the soft palate. The passage to the nasal cavity is free. The oral cavity is markedly large, and the throat cavity measures 18 mm.

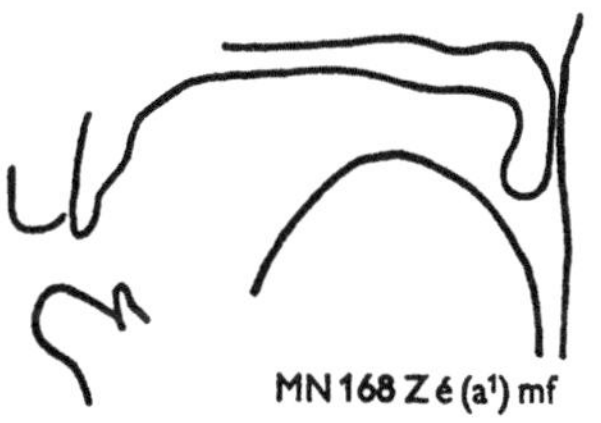

Fig. 21. Sung *é* (a^1) mf, MN 168, s. The lips are 10 mm apart. The tip of the tongue is drawn back such as to free the front part of the oral cavity. The tongue achieves maximal arching in the rear section of its crest; it approaches the soft palate to a distance of 11 mm. The velopharyngeal closure is unstable. On picture 168 a narrow gap is visible, on 169 there is a fine broken contact. The width of the throat cavity is particularly narrow in respect to its usual form.

[13] Viz e.g. analysis of shot 166 Z – 2,3 cm – fig. 10; 240 Š – 2,6 cm – fig. 19; contrast MN 160 where the speech-organs have a quite extraordinary form.

[14] On pictures 166 – fig. 10 *í* Z the closure is 15 mm long, on 271 – fig. 11 it is 6 mm long. When the distance is in excess of 20 mm (i.e. the width of the throat cavity at the root of the tongue) it is necessary that the soft palate with the uvula and the rear wall of the pharynx actively cooperate in forming the velopharyngeal closure.

[15] The front part of the oral cavity in test subject RV shows a severalfold increase, in RJ a twofold increase and in MN and LŠ a more than twofold increase, if we compare its size during the sung vowels *í* and *é*.

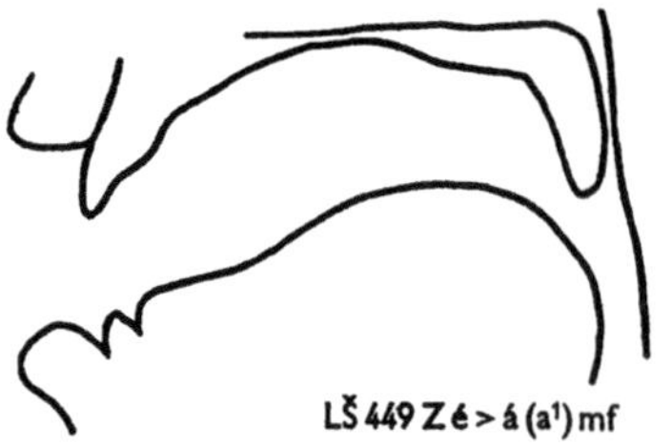

Fig. 22. Sung *é* (a^1) mf, LŠ 449, p. The intended *é* was very strongly coloured towards *á*. The distance between the lips measures 30 mm. The crest of the tongue is slightly dented in its front part. It continues obliquely upwards and is mildly arched in the rear section. The soft palate has moderate tonus and its upper contour is almost straight. The passage to the nasal cavity remains open.

In the majority of cases muscle-tension of the tongue can be described as moderate, the crest of the tongue only moderately arched towards the soft palate, almost the same as during *á*, though the root of the tongue is thrust forward, so that the throat cavity is smaller as against *í*, but almost twice as great as against *á*.[16] The tip of the tongue is either behind the lower incisors, or slightly raised and directed towards the gap between the lips. (figs. 23, 24, 25, 26.)

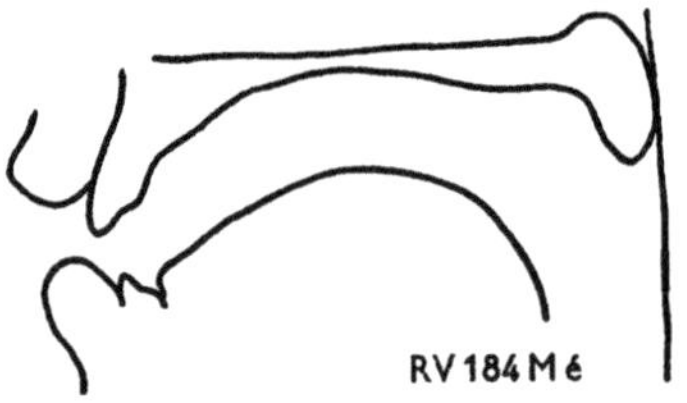

Fig. 23. Spoken *é* RV 184, s. The lips are 8 mm apart. The tip of the tongue is behind the lower incisors; the crest of the tongue is mildly arched and 16 mm away from the hard palate. The soft palate has tonus, is thickened and lightly touches the rear wall of the throat. The throat cavity measures 15 mm.

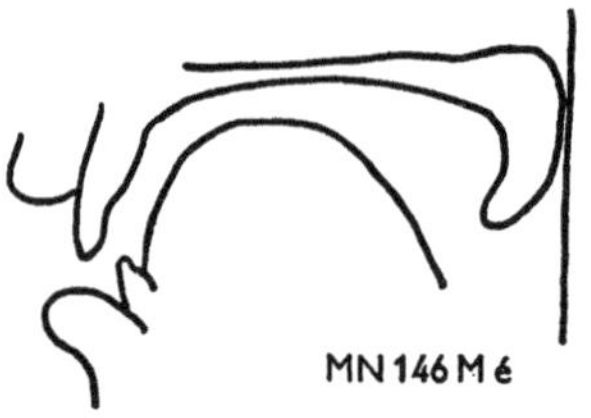

Fig. 24. Spoken *é* MN 146, s. The lips are 15 mm apart. The contour of the tongue is markedly similar to that during spoken *í*. The oral cavity is 0,25 its width during sung *é*. The summit of the crest of the tongue is a mere 5 mm away from the hard palate. The soft palate has tonus, and the uvula is pointed towards the oral cavity. Between the rear wall of the throat and the rear face of the soft palate there is a hairbreadth gap. The width of the throat cavity is considerably wider than with *é* sung by the same person.

[16] The width of the throat cavity fluctuates during sung *é* from 10 to 20 mm, while with sung *á* it does not exceed 10 mm.

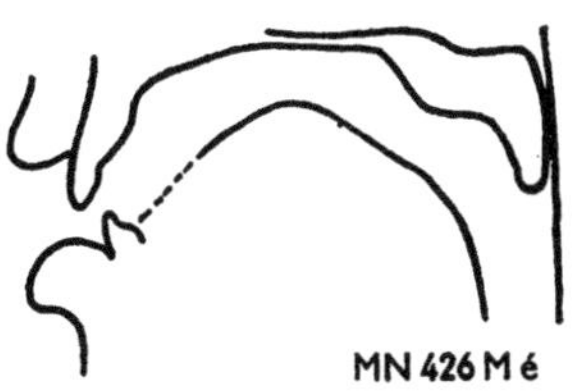

Fig. 25. Spoken *é* MN 426, s. The labial gap measures 11 mm. The tongue is in an irregular arch. The soft palate has an unusual form. It is indeed arched upwards in its rear section, but further forward it is indented. The peculiar bending of the upper contour of the soft palate is followed by a similar bending of its lower contour. The arch of the soft palate is 3 mm below the level of the plane of where the hard palate changes to the soft palate. The passage to the nasal cavity is closed. The width of the throat cavity measures 10 mm, which is more than twice the width during *é* sung by the same person.

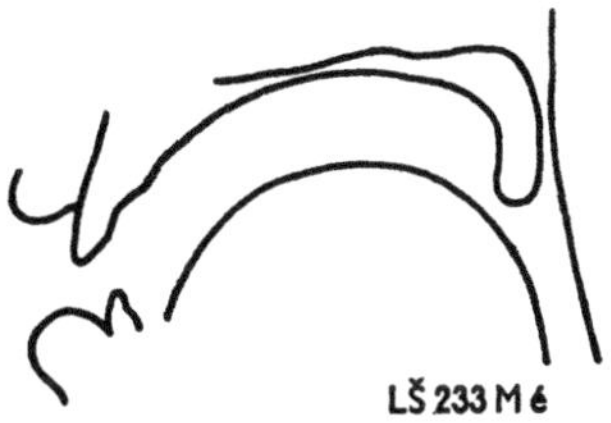

Fig. 26. Spoken *é* LŠ 233, s. The labial aperture is 15 mm wide. The tip of the tongue is behind the lower incisors. The regularly arched crest of the tongue is 14 mm away from the hard palate. The soft palate is very weakly tonized. It is raised and reaches the level of the hard palate by its upper contour. The passage to the nasal cavity remains free. The throat cavity measures 8 mm.

The size of the gap between the lips during the articulation of sung *é* is not noticeably greater than during spoken *é*; in some of the test subjects (e.g. RV, VM) it is even widest in whispered *é*. The size of the gap however during sung *é* changes in some cases in the same test subject. In comparison with the size of the labial gap during articulation of sung *í* the gap during sung *é* is almost twofold. (figs. 27, 28.)

The tonus of the soft palate can be observed in all cases, though it can be designated as weak. It is manifested by a raising of the soft palate to the level of the hard palate. In the majority of cases there is a velopharyngeal passage (of a width of 0.5-3 mm).

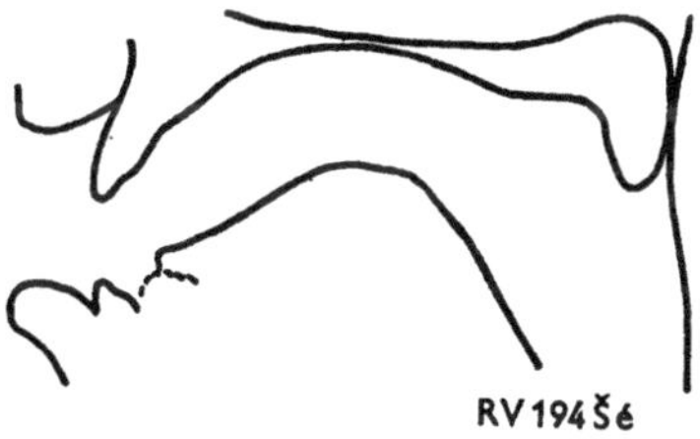

Fig. 27. Whispered *é* RV 194, s. The lips are 25 mm apart. The lower jaw is slightly thrust forward. The tip of the tongue touches the lower incisors. The tongue in the front section of the crest is slightly curved in. Its shape indicates marked tonus. The tonus of the soft palate is not very great; the soft palate touches the rear wall of the throat lightly. The width of the throat cavity measures 25 mm.

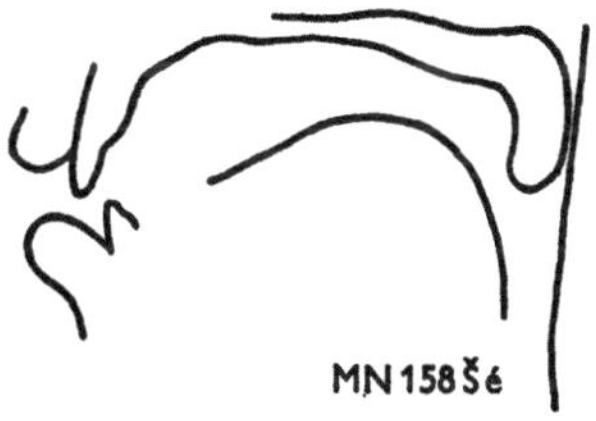

Fig. 28. Whispered *é* MN 158, s. The lips are 7 mm apart. The tongue is drawn back to the rear part of the oral cavity. The upper contour of the arching of the soft palate tends upwards, though it remains below the level of the plane of the hard palate. The tonus of the soft palate is very weak which corresponds to the articulatory stereotype of this test subject. The passage to the nasal cavity remains open. The throat cavity is 10 mm wide.

In some of the test subjects the velopharyngeal closure is quite unstable during sung *é* and changes during phonation.[17] On the other hand during *é* spoken and whispered the closure is more frequent.[18]

3. THE SPEECH ORGANS DURING THE ARTICULATION OF THE VOWEL *á*

During the realisation of sung *á* the front oral cavity enlarges either by the tongue being moved downward in the front part and backward in the rear part (in com-

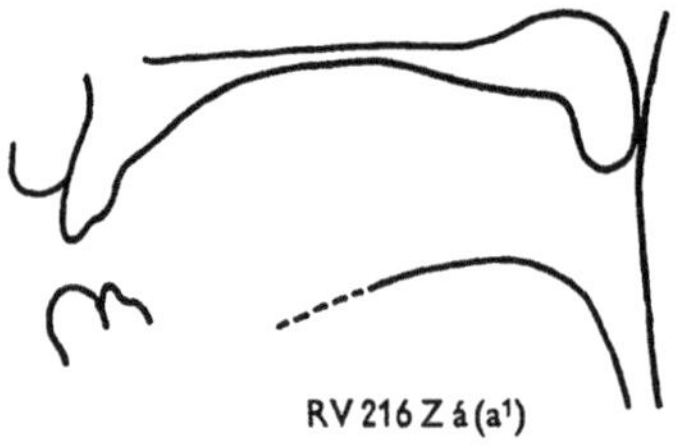

Fig. 29. Sung *á* (a1) pp, RV 216, s. The lips are 15 mm apart. The tongue lies most freely behind the teeth and is only mildly tonized. The muscular tension of the soft palate is marked. The soft palate is arched up above the level of the hard palate. On picture 216 it only makes contact with the rear wall of the throat, while on 217 it leaves a free passage to the nasal cavity. The throat cavity is 4 mm wide.

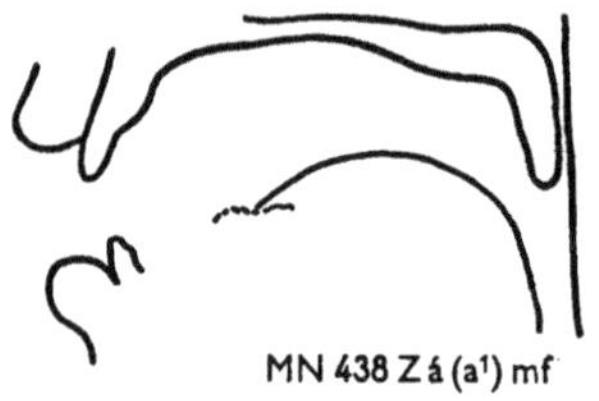

Fig. 30. Sung *á* (a1) mf, MN 438, s. The lips are 18 mm apart. The tongue is thrust back, is slightly arched and has no great tonus. The soft palate has very weak muscular tension. Over the whole length of its rear face is the passage to the nasal cavity. The throat cavity is 5 mm wide.

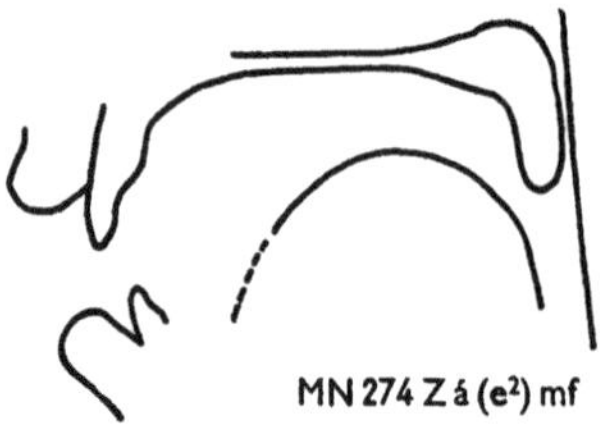

Fig. 31. Sung *á* (e2) mf, MN 274, s. The distance between the lips measures 17 mm. The tip of the tongue points to the lower incisors but does not touch them. The arch of the tongue approaches the uvula. There is mild tonus on the soft palate which does not touch the rear wall of the throat. The throat cavity measures 8 mm across.

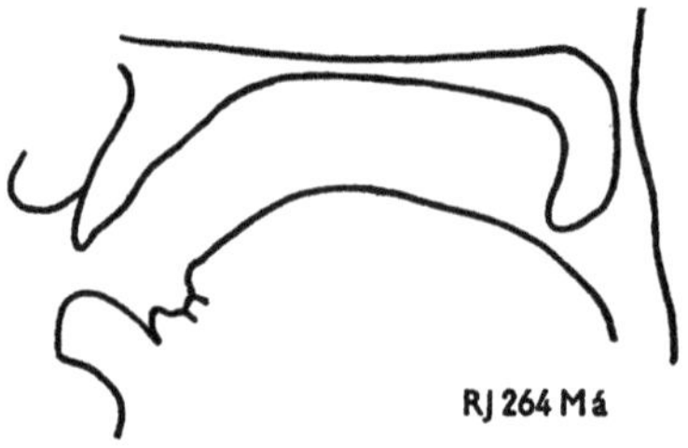

Fig. 32. Spoken *á* RJ 264, s. The lips are 15 mm apart. The tongue-tip rests against the lower incisors. The contour of the front part of the crest of the tongue slopes obliquely down to the tip. The rear half of the crest slopes more gently down to the root. The soft palate has only a little tonus and its upper contour remains on a level with the hard palate. The passage to the nasal cavity is open over the whole length of the rear face of the soft palate.

17 Most striking in MD; a 12 mm long closure alternates with a 1 mm wide passage.
18 With the spoken vowels it occurred four times out of ten, whispered – twice out of five.

parison with spoken *á*) when the jaw angle and labial gap remain approximately the same, or the labial gap is widened with an increase in the angle of the jaws. While during the realisation of spoken *á* there is in a large degree equilibrium between the sizes of the oral and throat cavities, during the articulation of sung *á* the oral cavity is enlarged. (figs. 29, 30, 31, 32.)

The tongue of the majority of cases has moderate tonus. During sung *á* it is moved some way backwards.

The tonus of the soft palate can be designated as very weak or moderate. However the soft palate is nevertheless raised to the level of the hard palate. The velopharyngeal closure was demonstrated in only two cases.[19] In three cases the closure was unstable;

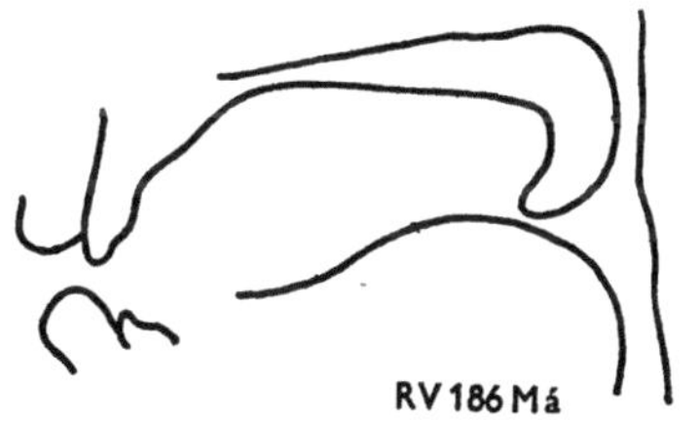

Fig. 33. Spoken *á* RV 186, s. The lips close up to 6 mm apart. The front part of the crest of the tongue is slightly dipped. The soft palate is mildly tonized. The uvula tends obliquely into the oral cavity. Passage to the nasal cavity remains open. The throat cavity is 7 mm wide.

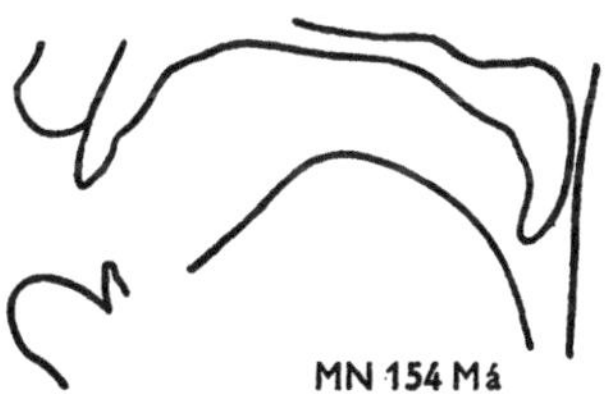

Fig. 34. Spoken *á* MN 154, s. The lips are 23 mm apart. The tongue is in an irregular upward arch, its summit being 15 mm from the hard palate. The soft palate is lowered and has a strongly undulating upper contour. The passage to the nasal cavity is free over the whole length of the rear face of the soft palate and the uvula. The throat cavity measures 7 mm across.

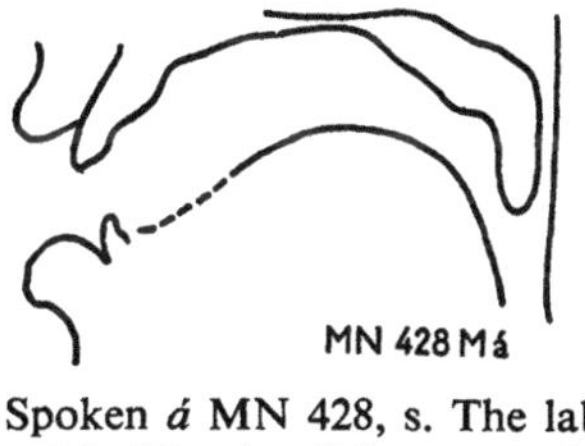

Fig. 35. Spoken *á* MN 428, s. The labial gap is 15 mm wide. The tip of the tongue is behind the lower incisors. The crest of the tongue reaches its summit in the central portion. The soft palate with the uvula hangs down, and its upper contour sinks below the level of the hard palate. The contour of its rear face is parallel with the rear wall of the throat. The passage to the nasal cavity remains open. The throat cavity measures 5 mm across.

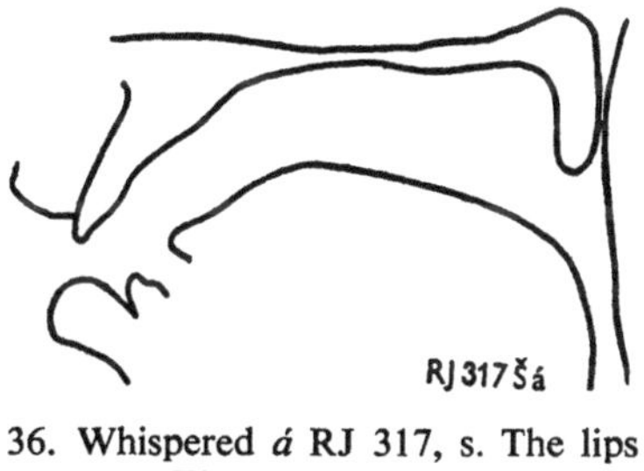

Fig. 36. Whispered *á* RJ 317, s. The lips are 12 mm apart. The tongue has mild tonus and its crest has a slightly broken contour. The upper outline of the soft palate is arched well above the level of the hard palate. The uvula points to the throat cavity. Between the soft palate and the rear of the throat there is a hairbreadth gap. The throat cavity measures 4 mm across.

[19] In RV – 4 mm, in MD – 3 mm.

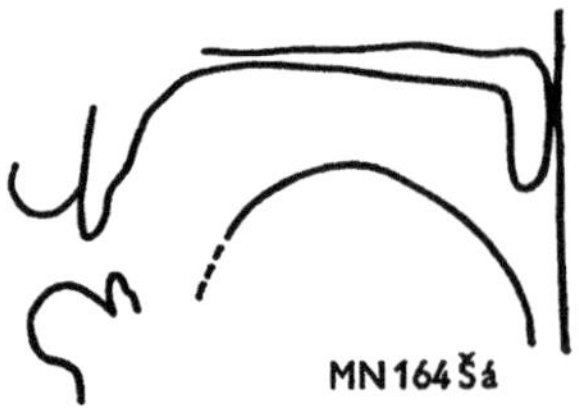

Fig. 37. Whispered *á* MN 164. The distance between the lips measures 12 mm. The tongue is arched and thrust to the back part of the oral cavity. The soft palate is in the same plane as the hard palate. The passage to the nasal cavity is lightly closed. The throat cavity is as with spoken *á*.

in nine cases there was a relatively narrow passage; in a further three the passage was significantly narrowed.[20] In no case however was the realised vowel *á* audially evaluated as nasal. (figs. 33, 34, 35, 36, 37.)

During spoken and whispered *á* the number of velopharyngeal closures and passage was in the same ratio as during sung *á*. However the velopharyngeal passage during spoken and whispered *á* was almost twice as wide as against sung *á*.

4. THE SPEECH-ORGANS DURING THE ARTICULATION OF THE VOWEL *ó*

During the articulation of sung *ó* the tongue is most arched at the rear part of its

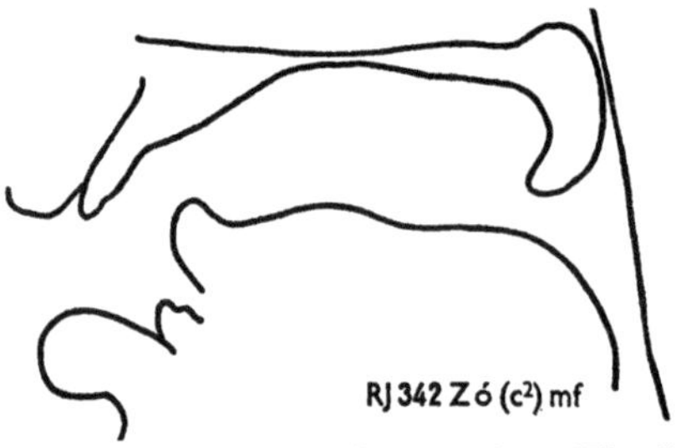

Fig. 38. Sung *ó* (c^2) mf, RJ 342, s. The lips are 18 mm apart. The tongue has strong tonus and is raised overall. The highest point of the tongue is its tip which is turned markedly up towards the alveolae. It is 10 mm away from them. The under-face of the tongue tip is opposite the labial aperture. The middle of the tongue crest is mildly dipped. The tonus of the soft palate is manifested in the fact that it is raised above the level of the hard palate and that the uvula points towards the oral cavity. The passage to the nasal cavity remains open. The throat cavity measures 8 mm across.

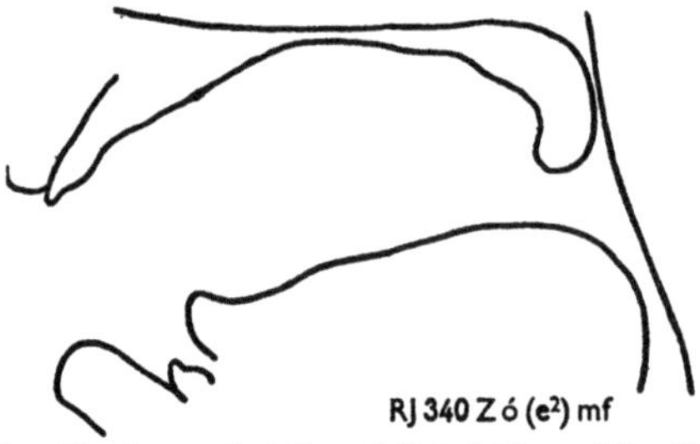

Fig. 39. Sung *ó* (e^2) mf RJ 340, s. The lips are 31 mm apart. The tongue has strong tonus though it remains on the floor of the oral cavity. The tip of the tongue points up towards the alveolae though it only goes as far as the lower lip. It is 40 mm from the alveolae. The front part of the crest of the tongue is gently undulated. The soft palate is at the level of the hard palate; it does not have any great muscular tension. The passage to the nasal cavity is open. In the area of the root of the tongue the throat cavity is 8 mm wide.

[20] In RJ, RV, and MN the pharyngeal passage during the realisation of sung *á* narrows by approximately a half in comparison with spoken *á*.

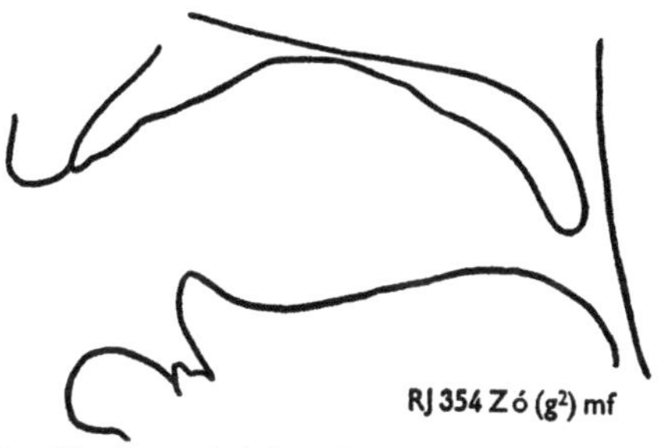

Fig. 40. Sung *ó* (g²) mf, RJ 354, s. The lips are 35 mm apart. The tip of the tongue points up and is 40 mm away from the alveolae. The central part of the crest of the tongue is slightly dipped. The soft palate leaves an open passage to the nasal cavity 5 mm wide. It is relaxed and does not reach the level of the hard palate. It resembles the soft palate with the mouth open and without phonation. The uvula points to the throat cavity which measures 6 mm across.

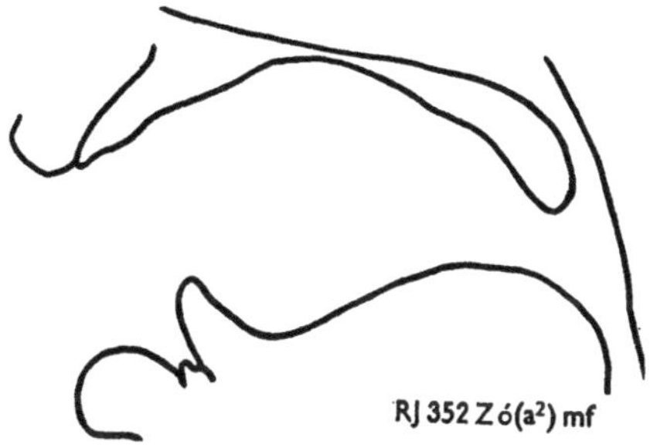

Fig. 41. Sung *ó* (a²) mf, RJ 352, s. The lips are 40 mm apart. The tongue has very strong tonus. However only the tip is raised and that 20 mm above the lower incisors. In spite of being thus raised the distance between its uppermost edge and the alveolae is 40 mm. The soft palate has a similar form to that when the mouth is open and without phonation. The passage to the nasal cavity is open. The throat cavity is 7 mm wide.

crest. This arching reduces through spoken *ó* towards whispered *ó* where there is only moderate arching of the tongue in the rear part of the crest. (figs. 38, 39, 40, 41.)

The throat cavity is narrower during sung *ó* than during spoken or whispered *ó*.

The labial gap is greatest during sung *ó*, decreases with spoken *ó* and is smallest during whispered *ó*.[21] It was possible to observe that the size of the labial gap also

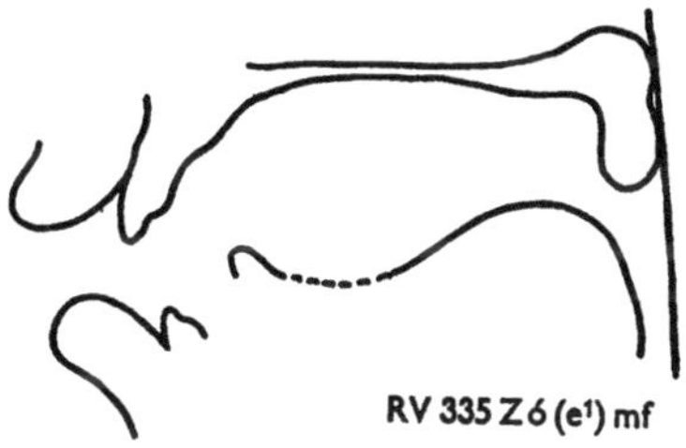

Fig. 42. Sung *ó* (e¹) mf, RV 335, s. On picture 334 the lips are 15 mm apart, and on 335 they are 12 mm apart. The tongue has marked tonus. The tip of the tongue is turned up and thrust forward so that it points towards the upper incisors. The central part of the tongue crest is dipped down and the rear part is arched up to 4 mm away from the uvula. The soft palate closes the passage to the nasal cavity by an interrupted contact with the rear wall of the throat. The throat cavity is 5 mm wide.

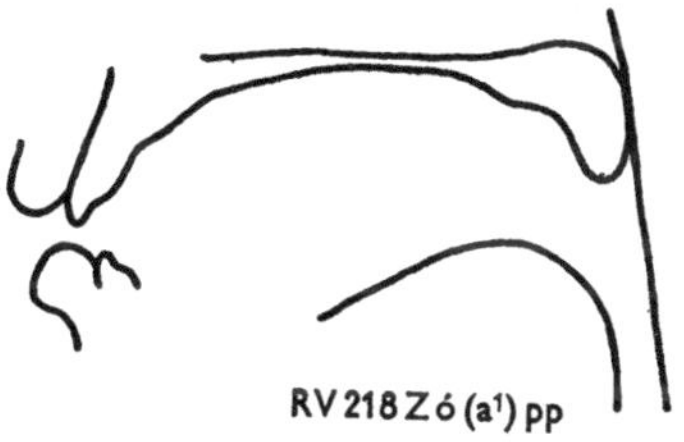

Fig. 43. Sung *ó* (a¹) pp, RV 218, s. The lips close to a distance of 4 mm. The tongue arches up very gently in the rear part of its crest. The muscular tension of the soft palate is very strong. The closure made by the soft palate with the rear wall of the throat is firm. The throat cavity measures 6 mm.

[21] In one subject only was the width of the labial gap in all cases of *ó* sung, spoken and whispered roughly the same; in one case during sung *ó* the lip gap was even narrower by two thirds than with spoken *ó*.

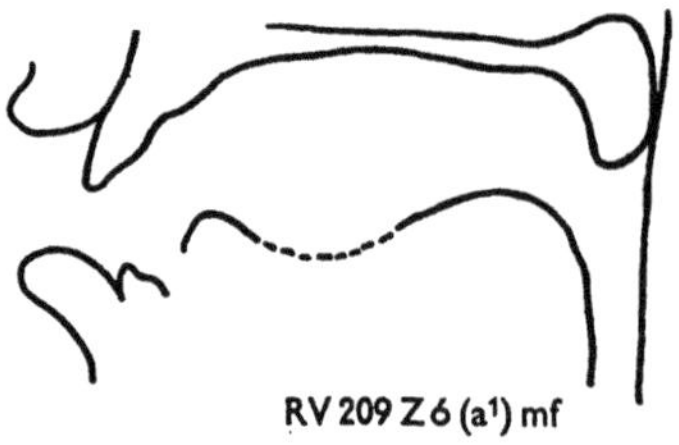

Fig. 44. Sung *ó* (a^1) mf, RV 209, s. The lips are 18 mm apart. The tip of the tongue points upwards. The crest of the tongue is dipped and in its rear section it is arched upwards to a distance of 20 mm from the soft palate. The tonus of the soft palate is strong, and its upper contour is strongly arched above the level of the hard palate. The passage to the nasal cavity is closed. The throat cavity measures 7 mm across.

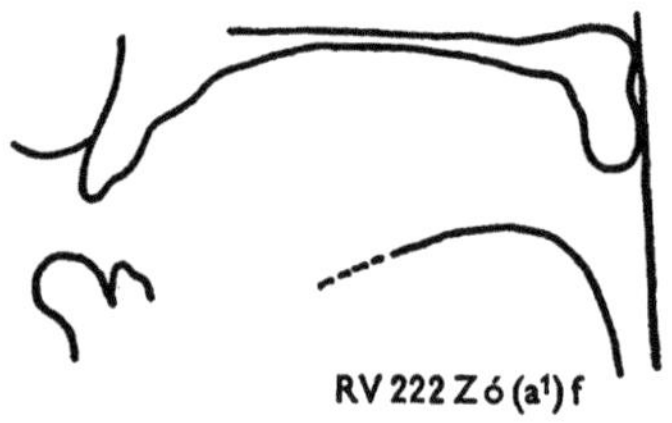

Fig. 45. Sung *ó* (a^1) f, RV 222, s. The lips are 17 mm apart. The tongue is tonized, lies low in the oral cavity and is drawn back. The tonus of the soft palate is marked. The soft palate makes interrupted contact with the rear wall of the throat. Its upper contour is only mildly arched above the level of the hard palate. The throat cavity is 5 mm wide.

increases when the vowel *ó* is realised at a higher tone.[22] Also the jaw angle is at its greatest during sung *ó* and again is greater at a higher tone, with which is of course connected the size of the labial gap.[23] (figs. 42, 43, 44, 45.)

According to the outline of the tongue on the X-ray picture, its tonus in all cases of sung *ó* is very strong, although not identically so in each individual test subject. In the professional singers as a result of great muscular tension the tip of the tongue is upraised, in one person with every case of sung *ó*, and in the remainder with *ó* sung at higher tones. As a result of the growing strength of the tone however, the tip of the tongue was not raised. In another case tonus of the tongue was manifested by greater arching. In non-singers the tongue has much greater tonus during sung *ó* and is also much more arched up towards the rear upper part of the oral cavity than during spoken and whispered *ó*. The tip of the tongue is not raised; it is drawn back and frees the forepart of the oral cavity as during spoken *ó*. During whispered *ó* however the tip of the tongue remains behind the lower incisors. It is possible to observe that in singers the position of the crest of the tongue in the oral cavity is proportionately lower as the tone is higher at which *ó* is sung. By this lowering of the tongue crest the capacity of the oral cavity is increased. On the other hand during spoken and whispered *ó* the arching of the rear part of the tongue crest is noticeably

22 This difference may be very great. In one subject we found a span of between 14 and 44 mm with *ó* sung at various pitches.

23 With the exception of one case (test subject MN) where the velopharyngeal closure was established twice with sung *ó* while with spoken and whispered *ó* the passage to the nasal cavity remains open. In two cases (one of a singer, one a nonsinger) there was always a free passage to the nasal cavity with spoken and whispered *ó*. In one case there was a clear free passage to the nasal cavity during spoken *ó*, and only during whispered *ó* was there contact between the soft palate and the rear wall of the pharynx. In the realisation of the professional singer there was a velopharyngeal closure during spoken and whispered *ó*.

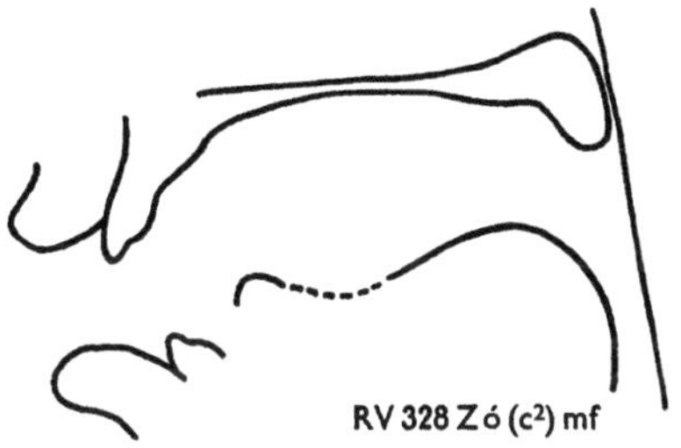

Fig. 46. Sung *ó* (c^2) mf, RV 328, s. The labial gap measures 20 mm. The tongue is saucer shaped which indicates strong tonus. It is dipped in its middle section. The tip points up to the alveolae. The rear section of the crest of the tongue is also arched up. The soft palate has marked tonus, though it leaves the passage to the nasal cavity open. The throat cavity measures 7 mm across.

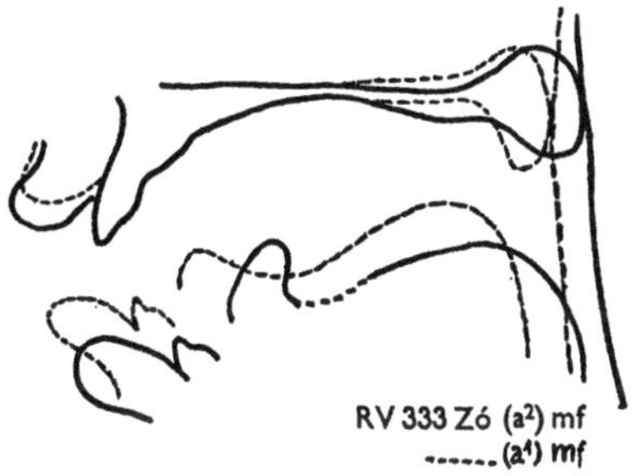

Fig. 47. Sung *ó* (a^2) mf, RV 333, s. The lips are 20 mm apart. In a forwards direction the crest of the tongue is drawn down in a dip. The tip is turned up and points backwards. The tonus of the tongue is very strong. The soft palate is unusually thickened at the lower outline of the uvula, and is strongly upraised. The upper contour of the soft palate rises sharply over the level of the hard palate. The passage to the nasal cavity is very firmly closed. The throat cavity measures 5 mm across.

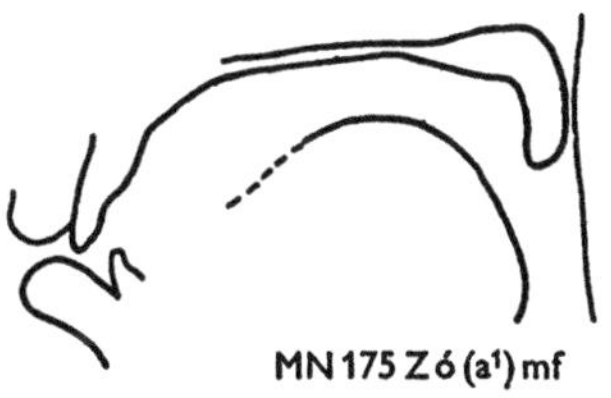

Fig. 48. Sung *ó* (a^1) mf, MN 175, s. The distance between the lips measures a mere 3 mm. The crest of the tongue is arched towards the soft palate to a distance of 10 mm. There is very weak tonus on the soft palate. Its upper contour is almost level. The passage to the nasal cavity is open. The throat cavity measures 11 mm across.

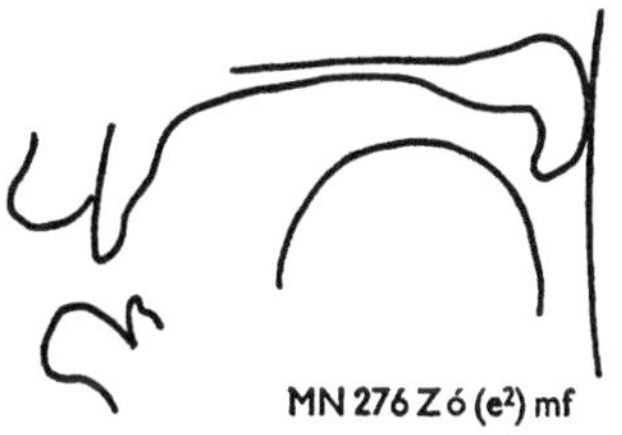

Fig. 49. Sung *ó* (e^2) mf, MN 276, s. The labial gap is 12 mm wide. The tip of the tongue points towards the floor of the oral cavity, approximately half-way back. The summit of the arch of the tongue crest is thrust further backwards and upwards in contrast to the articulatory shape during *ó* sung on a^1. The soft palate betrays marked tonus, though it only lightly touches the rear wall of the throat. The throat cavity is 7 mm wide.

less in singers. The tip of the tongue is not raised and during whispered *ó* is behind the lower incisors even in singers. (figs. 46, 47, 48, 49.)

We judge by its shape that the tonus of the soft palate is not very strong during sung *ó*. The velopharyngeal passage to the nasal cavity is on the whole wider than during spoken and whispered *ó*. In some singers the soft palate is even lowered during sung *ó* as its tonus is minimal. During spoken *ó* the tonus of the soft palate is somewhat stronger so that the soft palate is raised and only with whispered *ó* does the soft palate have strong tonus when it is fattened and touches the rear wall of the

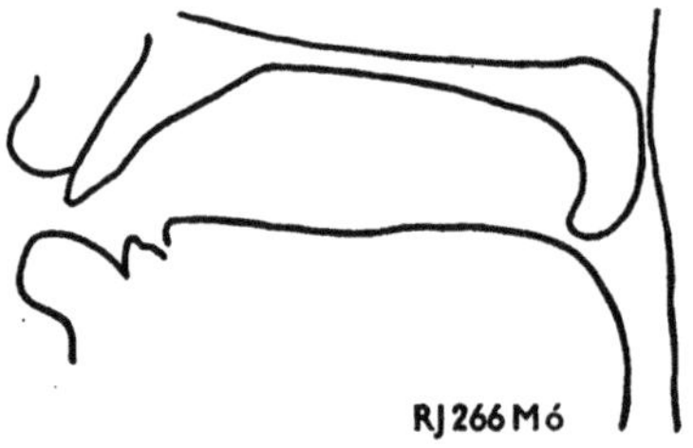

Fig. 50. Spoken *ó* RJ 266, s. The lips are 9 mm apart. The contour of the crest of the tongue remains almost level, with only a very slight tendency to rise towards the root of the tongue. The middle section of the tongue is trough-shaped lengthwise. The soft palate is tonized and the uvula bends in a crescent into the oral cavity; it comes very close to the rear part of the root of the tongue. The passage to the nasal cavity remains open.

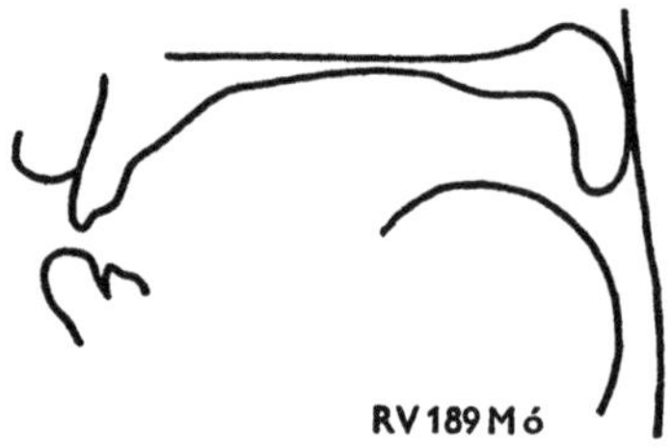

Fig. 51. Spoken *ó* RV 189, s. The distance between the lips measures 10 mm. The muscular tension of the tongue is indicated by the strong arching of the rear part of its crest in a direction backwards and upwards towards the uvula. The soft palate is raised well up and firmly closes the passage to the nasal cavity. The throat cavity measures 4 mm across.

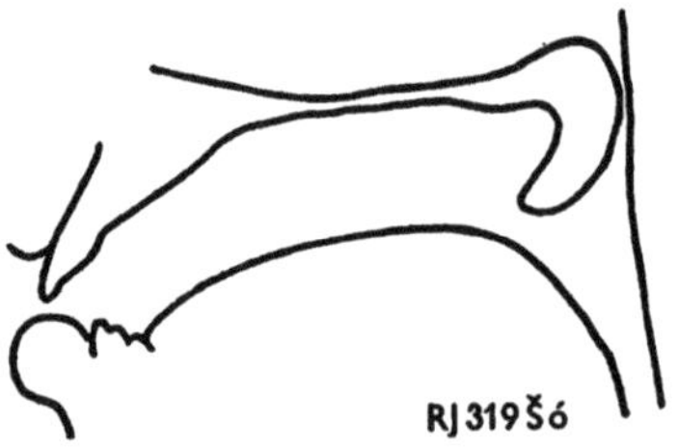

Fig. 52. Whispered *ó* RJ 319, s. The lips are 10 mm apart. The tip of the tongue is behind the lower incisors. The contour of the crest of the tongue rises gently towards its rear section. The soft palate has strong tonus, its upper contour is arched and the uvula points towards the oral cavity. The passage to the nasal cavity remains open. The throat cavity measures 6 mm across.

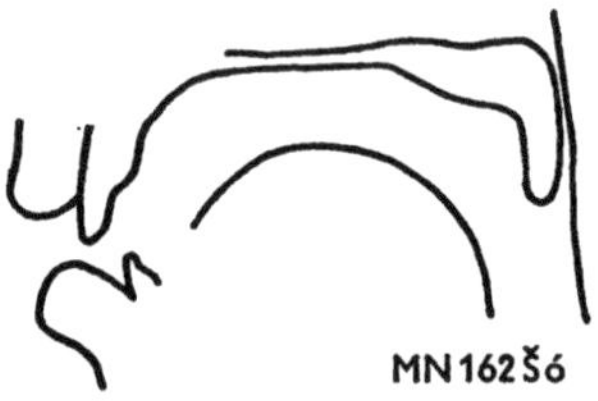

Fig. 53. Whispered *ó* MN 162, s. The labial aperture is 8 mm wide. The peak of the markedly arched crest of the tongue has moved somewhat forward so as to be pointing towards the hard palate from which it is 12 mm distant. The soft palate has weak tonus. Its upper contour with the exception of a slight dip is held at the level of the hard palate. The uvula points into the throat cavity. The passage to the nasal cavity remains open. The throat cavity is 15 mm wide.

throat. During the singing of *ó* one can clearly detect a gradual widening of the velopharyngeal passage from the low tones up to the high ones. (figs. 50, 51, 52, 53.)

On roentgeonograms recording the realisation of sung *ó* at various pitches and with varying intensity the passage to the nasal cavity is clearly visible. Only in one case during the singing of the vowel *ó* at a medium pitch was a velopharyngeal closure established. A very firm closure is made during pianissimo singing, just as in singing *ó* at a relatively high tone.

5. THE SPEECH-ORGANS DURING THE ARTICULATION OF THE VOWEL *ú*

During sung *ú* the labial gap is between two and four times wider than during spoken *ú*. With a raising or intensification of the tone the labial gap during sung *ú* was widened.[24]

The front oral cavity is wider during sung *ú* than during spoken *ú*, during whispered and sung *ú* it is roughly equally wide.[25]

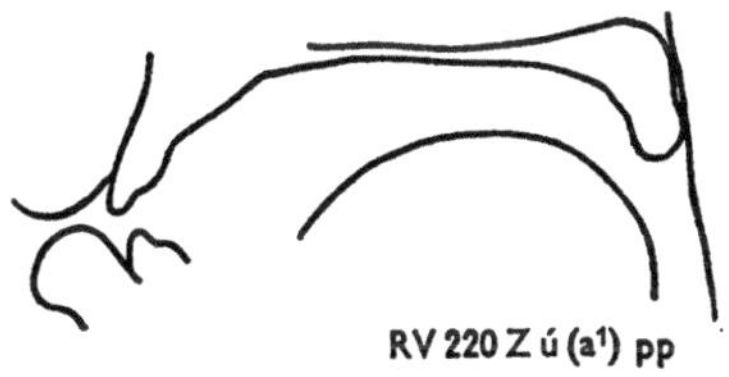

Fig. 54. Sung *ú* (a^1) pp, RV 220, s. The lips come as close as 2 mm apart. The tip of the tongue is drawn back on the floor of the oral cavity. The rear section of the crest of the tongue is mildly up-arched towards the back and is 7 mm from the soft palate. The tonus of the soft palate is stronger than during *ú* sung mezzoforte. On picture 220 there is clearly visible an interrupted contact of the uvula and the rear hanging face of the soft palate with the rear wall of the throat. The width of the throat cavity is 8 mm.

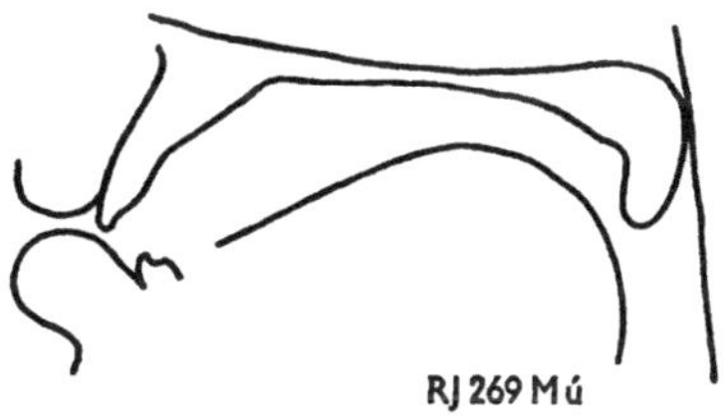

Fig. 55. Spoken *ú* RJ 269, s. The lips approach to 2 mm. The contour of the crest of the tongue slopes towards the tip. The peak of the tongue's arch is in the rear section of the crest. The tonus of the soft palate is greater than with sung *ú*. The rear face of the soft palate touches the rear wall of the throat. The throat cavity is 15 mm wide.

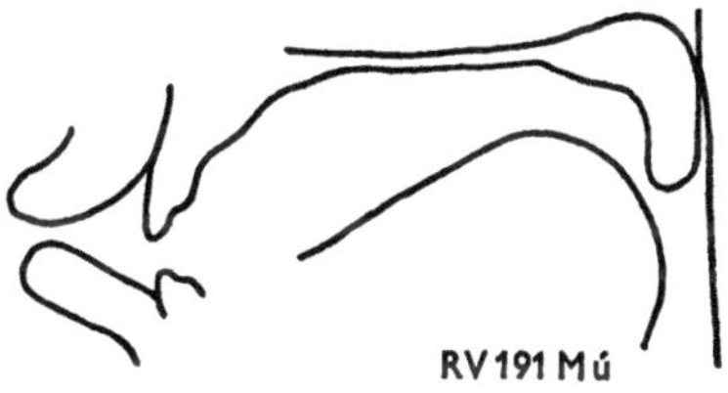

Fig. 56. Spoken *ú* RV 191, s. The lips are 3 mm apart. The arch of the crest of the tongue is backwards and upwards and approaches very close to the uvula. On picture 191 the passage to the nasal cavity is lightly closed, while on 190 there is a hairbreadth gap between the soft palate and the rear wall of the throat. The throat cavity measures 7 mm across.

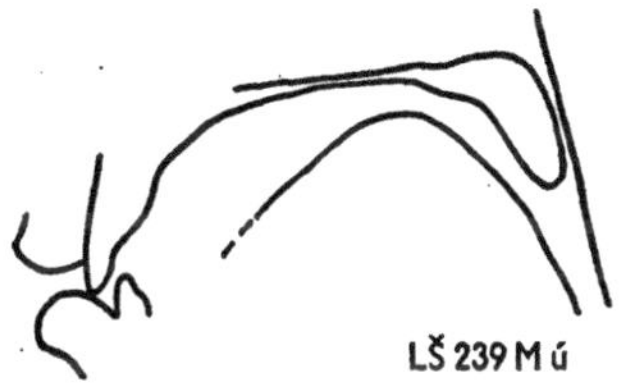

Fig. 57. Spoken *ú* LŠ 239, s. The lips are 3 mm apart. The crest of the tongue approaches the soft palate to a distance of 4 mm. The soft palate is lightly raised. The passage to the nasal cavity remains open. The throat cavity is 5 mm across.

[24] In test subject MN during spoken *ú* the labial aperture was as wide as during sung *ú* (with the exception of *ú* sung at the highest tone c^2 when the gap was as wide as during whispered *ú*). In this subject the gap was wider with whispered *ú* than with spoken *ú*.

[25] This information comes from the analysis of the speech-organs in articulation of test subjects RV and MN. In test subject LŠ no difference was to be seen in the width of the front oral cavity as between whispered *ú* and spoken *ú*. In test subject RJ the oral cavity was narrowest with spoken *ú*, it was wider with whispered *ú*, and with sung *ú* it was twice as large as with spoken *ú*.

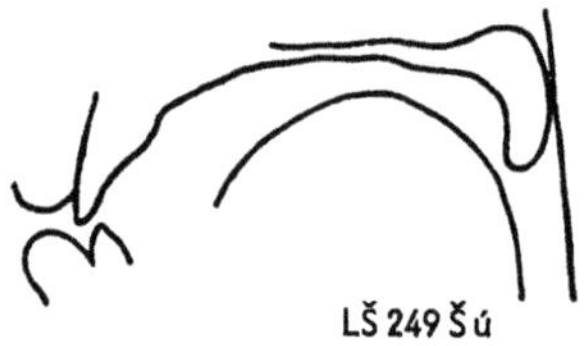

Fig. 58. Whispered *ú* LŠ 249, s. The lips are 3 mm apart. The tongue is arched backwards and upwards. The summit of its crest points towards the soft palate which lightly closes the passage to the nasal cavity by contact with the rear wall of the throat. The soft palate is mildly arched over the level of the hard palate.

In the forward-backward direction the tongue is pushed back and in the vertical direction is thrust upwards. In all cases the crest during sung *ú* is less upward arched than during spoken *ú*. In one case (test subject RJ) it was even level during sung *ú*. The tip of the tongue is drawn downwards during sung, spoken and whispered *ú*. In the majority of cases it lies on the floor of the mouth. In one case the tip of the tongue is raised and tends towards the alveolae; in a further case the tip is raised during spoken *ú* and tends towards the labial gap.

According to its outline on the roentgenograms the tonus of the tongue is in the majority of cases marked to strong. The tongue is thrust back and up, but less so during sung *ú* than with spoken *ú*. (figs. 54, 55, 56, 57, 58.)

The tonus of the soft palate is weak. The soft palate is always raised to the level of the hard palate; in some cases it is even fattened particularly when there is a velopharyngeal closure. During sung *ú* the velopharyngeal closure occurs only rarely. If the passage to the nasal cavity is closed there is merely contact between the rear wall of the soft palate and that of the throat. Also analyses of serial roentgenograms of the articulatory position of the speech-organs during sung *ú* show that it is an unstable contact which fluctuates even during tension of the vowel. Not even the passage to the nasal cavity is very large.[26] Out of thirteen cases the soft palate made contact with the rear wall of the pharynx seven times; in six cases the passage to the nasal cavity was free. Out of eighteen cases of spoken and whispered *ú* there were ten where there was a passage to the nasal cavity and eight where the soft palate made contact with the back wall of the throat. Neither during the photographing nor during the perception test against a sound recording was it possible to distinguish audially between the realisations with open or closed passage to the nasal cavity.

With a reduction of intensity of the sung vowel *ú* there was a noticeable reduction of width (size) of the rear oral cavity so that when *ú* was sung pianissimo the cavity was reduced by half in cross-section, while however the front oral cavity remained without change.

[26] In the majority of cases it is 0,5-1 mm wide; in isolated cases it may be as wide as 2-3 mm.

By the thrusting backwards and upwards of the tongue the width of the pharyngeal cavity changes; however this is quite individual and varies from person to person.

6. THE SPEECH-ORGANS DURING NEUTRAL NASAL AND ORAL SOUNDS AND WITHOUT PHONATION

From each test subject we analysed pictures of the speech organs during neutral nasal and oral sounds, and without phonation. The size of jaw angle, the labial gap and the oral cavity changes according as the mouth is open or closed. On the other hand there

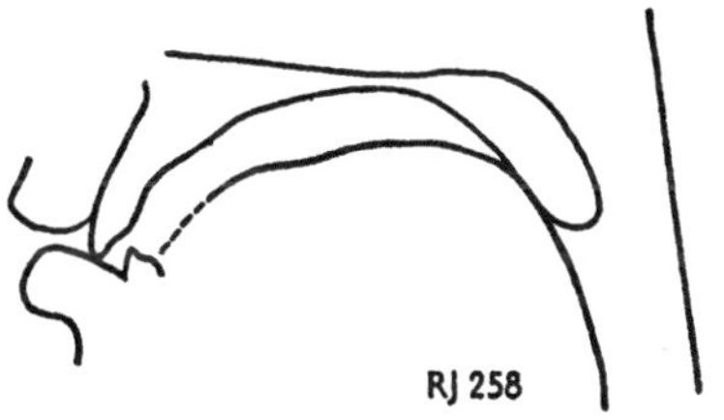

Fig. 59. Articulation of a neutral nasal sound, RJ 258, s. The lips are a mere 3 mm apart. The tip of the tongue is behind the lower incisors. Its crest is gently arched. The soft palate is lowered and touches the crest of the tongue. The passage to the nasal cavity measures 13 mm across.

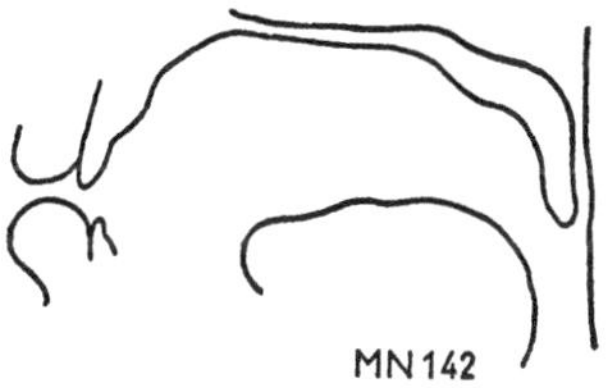

Fig. 60. Articulation of a neutral nasal sound, MN 142, s. There is a 2 mm gap between the lips. The tip of the tongue is drawn back. It remains however in the plane of the lower molars. The passage to the nasal cavity is only 2 mm wide. There is clearly detectable tonus of the soft palate. The mild arching of the soft palate begins 5 mm below the level of the hard palate, then the back contour of the uvula follows the rear wall of the throat in a parallel line. The uvula points into the throat cavity which is 10 mm wide.

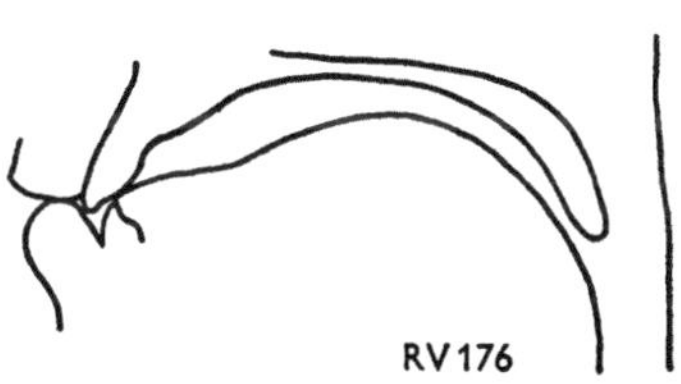

Fig. 61. The speech-organs without phonation – mouth closed – RV 176, s. The lips are closed. The tip of the tongue lies behind the upper incisors. The crest of the tongue is slightly undulated in its middle section. The rear section arches upwards towards the soft palate which is lowered but does not touch the rear part of the tongue crest. The passage to the nasal cavity is 10 mm wide as is the throat cavity also.

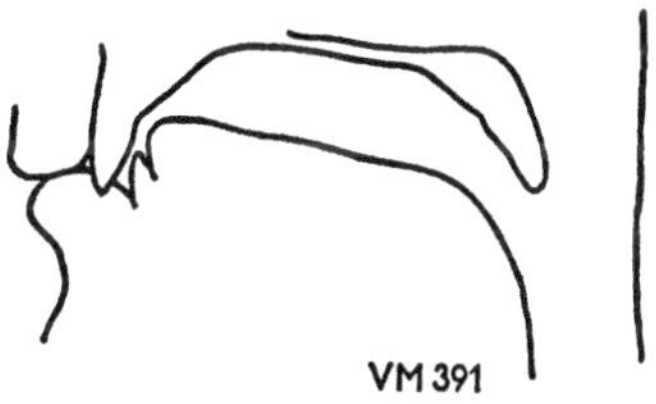

Fig. 62. The speech-organs without phonation – mouth closed – VM 391, s. The lips touch. The tip of the tongue is slightly raised and tends towards the alveolae from which it is 3 mm distant. From the tip the crest of the tongue slowly descends towards the tongue root. The soft palate remains in the plane of the hard palate. The passage to the nasal cavity is 16 mm wide. The uvula is protracted though it does not touch the root of the tongue. It points into the throat cavity whose width reaches 17 mm.

is no significant change in the relative positions of the tongue, the soft palate and the uvula, nor in the size of the pharyngeal passage. (figs. 59, 60.) The passage to the nasal cavity is open at maximum. In some cases the uvula almost touches the rear part of the crest of the tongue when the mouth is closed. (figs. 61, 62.)

When the mouth is open there is only very moderate tonus on the soft palate and the tongue. The contour of the root of the tongue is usually parallel to the back wall of the throat, and the distance between them may be taken as a basis for the evaluation of the other pictures. The soft palate is in some cases so lax that it touches the tongue with the uvula; in other cases the crest of the tongue and the uvula are further apart than on the pictures with the mouth closed, because with the mouth open the soft palate is raised. As a rule the soft palate is away from the back wall of the throat so that there is a clear velopharyngeal passage. The tongue is, at the rear part of the crest, arched upwards, its tip behind the lower incisors.[27]

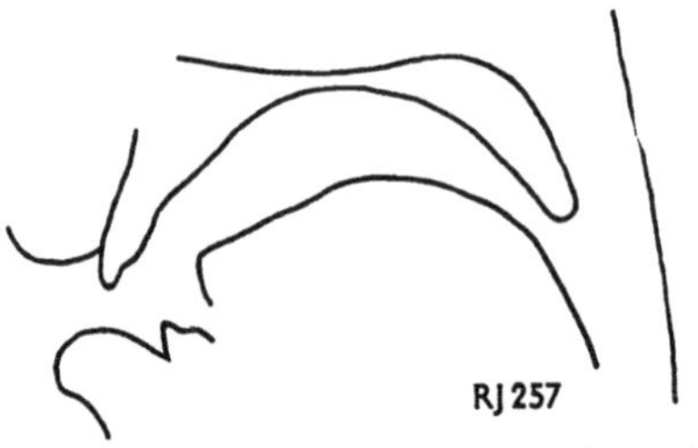

Fig. 63. The speech-organs without phonation – mouth open – RJ 257, s. The lips are 11 mm apart. The tip of the tongue is raised above the cutting edge of the lower incisors. The crest of the tongue is mildly arched. The soft palate is lowered though it makes no contact by the uvula with the root of the tongue. The passage to the nasal cavity in the region of the soft palate is 14 mm wide. The width of the throat cavity is also 14 mm.

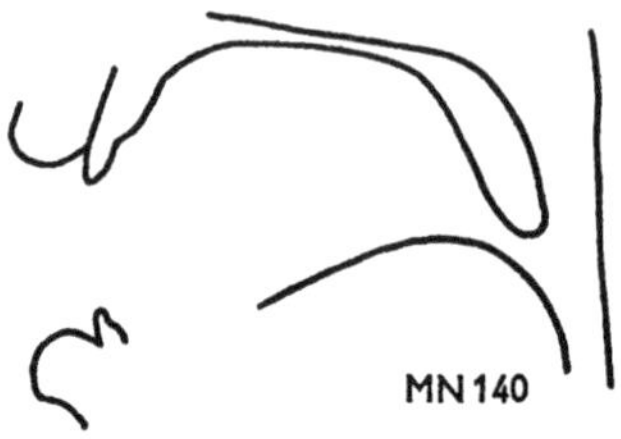

Fig. 64. The speech-organs without phonation – mouth open – MN 140, s. The labial gap is 27 mm wide. The tongue follows the slope of the lower jaw. The soft palate hangs freely down. The passage to the nasal cavity is 8 mm wide and the throat cavity is 6 mm wide.

By an analysis of roentgenograms of the speech-organs during a neutral nasal sound we discovered that the formation of the speech-organs corresponds to a large degree to the position without phonation. The passage to the nasal cavity is open, the soft palate lowered and the uvula in some cases almost touching the rear part of the crest of the tongue. (figs. 63, 64.)

On roentgenograms of the speech-organs during pronunciation of a neutral oral sound there is a clear velopharyngeal closure.

27 In test subject MN there is visible a clear movement of the soft palate and particularly the root of the tongue towards the rear wall of the throat.

IV

ANALYSES OF THE ARTICULATORY MOVEMENTS

As is clear from the preceding paragraphs most important material for the analysis of the action of the speech-organs was the cineradiographic sound film "The movement of the tongue and the soft palate in the singing of vowels". It contains three series of analogous shots.

Shots of the speech-organs without phonation with open and closed mouth were included (in the same way as when we were using static shots) in order that we might establish what movements were possible and habitual during articulation in each of the test subjects. Then come shots of the long spoken vowels pronounced once in the words *pít, péci, pád, pól, půl,* and once in isolation, in such a way that first was always pronounced the word with the vowel concerned so that then there was a natural situation for the utterance of the immediately following isolated vowel. The utterances were then thus: *pít – í, péci – é, pád – á, pól – ó, půl – ú.* Initial *p* as a bilabial non-nasal stop was chosen in order that we could identify with certainty the beginning of the phonation of each vowel.

Shots of the speech-organs during the sung vowels were taken in combination with the consonant *b* in the order *bí, bé, bá, bó, bú,* so that the vowels also follow a bilabial non-nasal stop this time voiced, and they correspond to the material obtained from serial roentgenography. Because even on the static pictures of the speech-organs during the singing of vowels at different frequencies there were indications of their distinctive articulation, we included in the film shots of the vowel sung at different pitches. The pitch was always established on the basis of the vocal range of the test subject and with a view to the critical tonal areas.[1] With each test subject we made a preliminary experiment to discover whether the desired tone would be suitable for him.

Next were included shots of the articulation of sung syllables at the same pitch f ♯^{1} 367-Hz for the first series, e^1 – 326 – Hz for the second series, and for the third series a♭ – 209 Hz, and with varying intensity.

[1] "Das Stimmgefüge einer Person ist das Gesamt der Noten, die ohne besondere Anstrengung hervorgebracht werden können. Bei einem Sänger mit sehr gepflegter und einwandfrei hervorgebrachter Stimme neigt das Gefüge dazu, den gesamten Stimmbereich einzunehmen, und zuweilen decken sich Gefüge und Gesamtstimmbereich tatsächlich. Wir unterlegen ihm daher diesen letzten Sinn." (R. Husson, "Der gegenwärtige Stand der physiologischen Phonetik", *Phonetica* 4 [1959] 12).

Because we had discovered from the material obtained by the methods used previously that the vowel *é* was the most complex as to its movements, and interesting in the instability of the velopharyngeal closure we included among the cineradiographic shots the phonation of this vowel in a bound sung scale, rising and falling.[2]

The second and third series were further supplemented by a detail picture of the area of the uvula during the bound sung scale, and by a plane shot with a moving camera from the lips over the tongue and the soft palate as far as the upper part of the larynx.

The shots were centered on the supraglottal cavities and record the movements of

[2] In the checking of the tonal pitches realised we had the very willing and devoted cooperation of Prof. A. Sychra, DrSc.

Three prop points were used to fix the head position of the test subjects in such a way that they could not move from the desired position. As the apparatus took in a circle of 13 cm diameter there was a danger that if the test subject moved at all, the whole area under investigation might not have been recorded.

The photographing of the cineradiographic shots by the complex method called for seven people in addition to the test subjects (i.e. roentgenologist, two phoneticians, two nurses, a cameraman and a laboratory assistant.) In making the cineradiographic recordings the desired pitch was given to the test subject by a tone generator. In the syllables sung at various pitches an average loudness was required. With the syllables sung at the same pitch the loudness was changed in the ranges pianissimo, mezzoforte and fortissimo. To ensure accurate relative reactions between the loudness of the individual syllables we also took records of the loudness level with a Brüel and Kjaer sound level recorder. Technical data: cut off frequency 80, potentiometer 50 dB, recording speed 70 mm, writing speed 3 mm. Lines indicate intervals of 5 dB. (viz. further figs. 65, 70, 73, 75, 78, 81, 82, 84, 85.)

The sound of the film camera was quite marked but was nevertheless well below the sound level of the sung syllables. In test subject RJ this difference was about 20 dB in syllables sung mezzoforte, at pianissimo it is about 15 dB and at fortissimo the smallest difference is 20 dB. There were also further differences in the specific loudness of the individual vowels. The vowels *a* and *o* are marked by a greater specific loudness than the remainder. Specific loudness of vowels and its relation to resultant loudness can be assessed only on the basis of the whole group sung during one set of shots, as during the next set there is usually a change in the overall voice intensity. (On specific loudness see P. Janota, "K otázce měření dynamiky řeči", thesis 1949.) During the analyses of the shots we discovered quite marked individual differences in the conception of the different degrees of tonal loudness. In test subject RA for instance fortissimo was separated from pianissimo by a range of from 8-40 dB; pianissimo from mezzoforte by from 2-12 dB, and between mezzoforte and fortissimo in the same subject there was a difference of from 2-32 dB. Test subject JH on the other hand showed a relatively small difference between pianissimo and mezzoforte (the weakest pianissimo and the strongest mezzoforte are separated by 9 dB.) The highest level of mezzoforte exceeded the lowest level of fortissimo by 1 dB and the difference between the weakest mezzoforte and the strongest fortissimo was only 6 dB. The level of loudness during the course of the ascending and descending sung scale is quite variable.

Of particular interest in the material are the transitional articulatory features which occur with the realisation of consonant and vowel in a syllable. The investigation of transitional features in phonetics is of great interest in Prague too as is shown e.g. by the works of M. Romportl and A. Skaličková. In view of the fact that this mentioned cineradiographic recording is the first recording of Czech sung, spoken and whispered vowels of this kind, it was appropriate to investigate the syllables separately, and the transitional phenomena only within the framework of the individual syllable. However it was not possible to eliminate from the test subjects preparation for the articulation of the next syllable. Articulatory preparation is frequently very clearly visible on the shots.

Before each shot was taken, all technical data were recorded on the synchronous sound record. These covered the number of the shot, the name of the test subject, the pitch and intensity of the realised syllable.

the tongue and the soft palate. No use was made of any contrast media. The edited and sub-titled sound film is 332 m long.[3]

The resulting analyses are given according to the individual shots recording the course of the articulation of syllables with the same initial consonant /*b*/ and different final vowels /*í, é, á, ó, ú*/, and give a comparison of the realisations of three test subjects (the first [RJ], second [RA] and third [JH] series).

1. THE SPEECH-ORGANS WITH THE MOUTH CLOSED

First series. The soft palate is free and far from the rear wall of the throat. It hangs down though it does not touch the tongue. Also there is no muscular tension of the tongue.

Second series. The soft palate is free though not without some degree of muscular tension. It touches the root of the tongue with only a small area of contact. The passage between the rear wall of the throat and the soft palate is not uniformly wide overall. Between the uvula and the rear wall of the throat the passage is much narrower than between the rear wall of the soft palate and the rear wall of the throat. The narrowing of this passage in the direction towards the throat cavity is emphasised by the oblique slope of the root of the tongue, if we consider the rear part of the crest

[3] The content of the film:

First series (RJ)

1. Shots of the movements of the articulatory organs during the spoken vowels in words, and shots of the isolated vowels *pít – í, péci – é, pád – á, pól – ó, půl – ú*. 2. Syllables sung with the same intensity and at the tonal pitch g ♯ – 204 Hz, in the order *bí, bé, bá, bó, bú*. 3. Syllables sung with the same intensity at the tonal pitch d^1 – 294 Hz. 4. Syllables sung with the same intensity at the tonal pitch f^1 – 348 Hz. 5. Syllables sung with the same intensity at the tonal pitch g $♯^1$ – 408 Hz. 6. Syllables sung at the same tonal pitch f $♯^1$ – 367 Hz pianissimo, mezzoforte and fortissimo. 7. The vowel *é* in the continuous scale of G major sung up and down.

Second series (RA)

1. Shots of the movements of the organs of articulation during spoken vowels in words and shots of the pronunciation of isolated vowels: *pít – í, péci – é, pád – á, pól – ó, půl – ú*. 2. The syllables *bí, bé, bá, bó, bú* sung with the same intensity at the tonal pitch f ♯ – 184 Hz. 3. The syllables sung with the same intensity at the tonal pitch c^1 – 261 Hz. 4. The syllables sung with the same intensity at the tonal pitch d $♯^1$ – 306 Hz. 5. The same syllables sung with the same intensity at the tonal pitch f $♯^1$ – 367 Hz. 6. The same syllables sung at the same tonal pitch e^1 – 326 Hz at intensities pianissimo, mezzoforte and fortissimo. 7. The vowel *á* sung up and down the continuous scale of F-major. 8. A shot of the vowel *é* in a continuous sung scale with a camera moving from the lips over the tongue and the soft palate to the upper part of the larynx.

Third series (JH)

1. Shots of the movements of the organs of articulation during spoken vowels in words and shots of the pronunciation of the isolated vowels: *pít – í, péci – é, pád – á, pól – ó, půl – ú*. 2. The syllables *bí, bé, bá, bó, bú* sung with the same intensity at the tonal pitch b ♭ – 232 Hz. 3. The same syllables sung with the same intensity at the tonal pitch f – 174 Hz. 4. The same syllables sung with the same intensity at the tonal pitch g ♯ – 204 Hz. 5. The same syllables sung with the same intensity at the tonal pitch b ♭ – 232 Hz. 6. The same syllables sung at the same tonal pitch a ♭ – 209 Hz with intensities pianissimo, mezzoforte and fortissimo. 7. The vowel *é* sung up and down in the continuous scale of A-major. 8. A shot from the lips to the lower part of the larynx.

of the tongue and the rear wall of the soft palate as continuous. Even with the mouth closed a certain muscular tension is detectable in the speech-organs although it is very weak. This shows that we cannot identify the notion 'speech-organs without phonation' with the notion 'speech-organs at rest'.

Third series. The soft palate hangs down and makes contact with the rear part of the crest and the root of the tongue.

2. THE SPEECH-ORGANS WITH THE MOUTH OPEN

First series. The soft palate is so free (in contrast to the position with the mouth closed) that the uvula touches the tongue. It is far from the rear wall of the throat.

Second series. The tongue at the rear part of the crest is arched upwards. The front part of the crest of the tongue is pulled forwards. The tip of the tongue is on the floor of the oral cavity. The width of the passage of the nasal cavity is almost uniform throughout. The crest of the tongue and the uvula are further apart than in the shot of the closed mouth, because the soft palate is raised. The shot finishes with a movement of the tongue; it is a movement downwards and backwards by which the tongue approaches the rear wall of the throat. At the same time the tongue remains well arched upwards. This shot of the open mouth in comparison to that of the closed mouth is an interesting proof of the active approach of the rear wall of the throat to the soft palate. Also participation of the throat wall which is manifested by its arching towards the soft palate, and its passive position without arching when the mouth is closed.

Third series. With open mouth the throat cavity is very narrow. The tongue comes downwards and backwards. The central part of the crest and the tip of the tongue are on the floor of the oral cavity. The soft palate is raised though a small velo-pharyngeal passage remains.

3. THE MOVEMENT OF THE ARTICULATORY ORGANS DURING THE SPOKEN VOWELS

First series. On the pictures are quite clear the muscular movements during the realisation of the individual spoken words and the individual vowels. The nerve impulse has as a result a very abrupt arching of the soft palate upwards. In the pronunciation of *pít* and the vowel *í* raising of the soft palate is at its greatest. In the other words and isolated vowel */péci – é, pád – á, pól – ó, půl – ú/*, the soft palate is freer.

Also during the movement of the tongue similar impulses are manifest. In the pronunciation of the syllable */pít/* with the vowel *í* the tongue goes upwards and forwards. During isolated *í* the tongue goes higher and further forward than in the preceding word. During *é* the tongue is less raised and during the remaining vowels

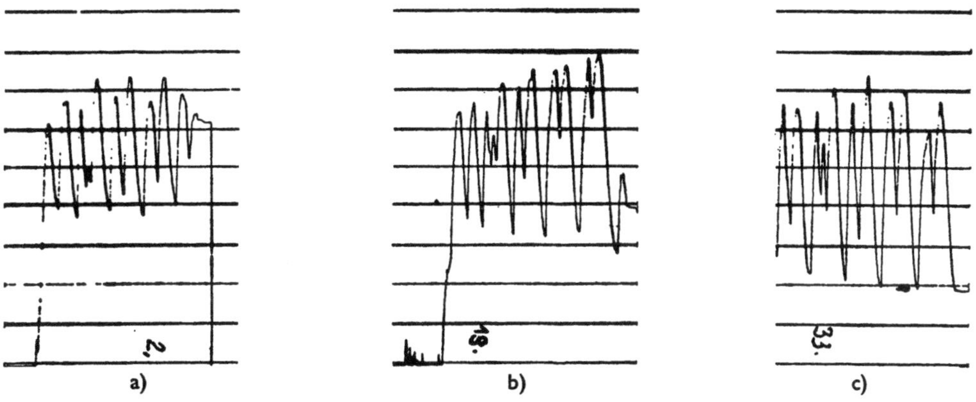

Fig. 65. Recording of the intensity of spoken words and vowels: *pít – í, péci – é, pád – á, pól – ó, půl – ú,* (a) 1st series, (b) 2nd series, (c) 3rd series.

/á, ó, ú/ it is, quite the reverse, thrust gradually downwards. During *ó* and *ú* the tongue is seen to be generally curved and at the same time undulating. The tongue arches rapidly backwards and upwards in its rear part and its contour is rounded. During the phonation of the word '*pól*' is just when we find this undalation, i.e. in the first movement phase the form of the rear part of the tongue is rounded and in the next phase the rounding is reduced and the tongue (fig. 66) stretches out more lengthwise in a forward direction though the rounded shape remains in a milder degree.[4]

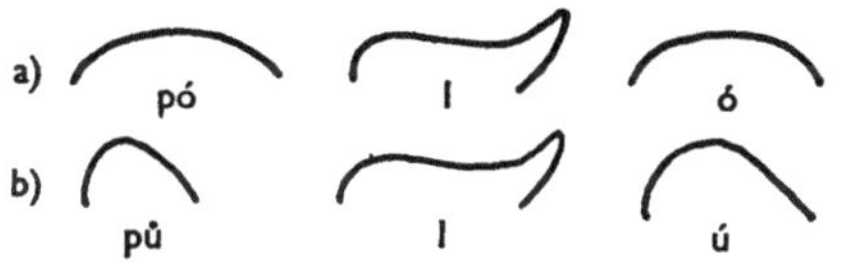

Fig. 66. Schematic representation of the movement of the tongue in the pronunciation of (a) *pól – ó*, (b) *půl – ú*. A definite dipping of the crest of the tongue occurs caused by the pronunciation of the consonant *l* between the vowels (lips to the right).

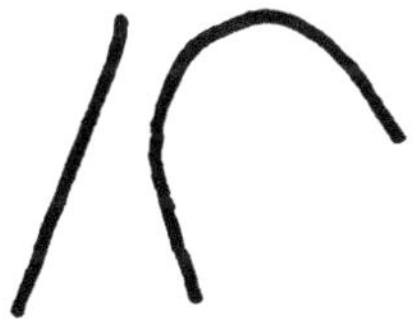

Fig. 67. Schematic representation of the shape of the throat cavity and the tongue during the pronunciation of *ú* in the word půl (2nd series – lips to the right).

[4] It is influenced by the articulation of the consonant *l* which is clearly visible on the shots of the word *pól* and *půl*. During the following *l* contact is made between the tongue and the hard palate. This gives the impression of a certain fluctuation which is emphasised in the pronunciation of the sequence *pól – ó, půl – ú*.

Second series. The whole concentration of the articulatory movements is shifted backwards (i.e. as far as the tongue is concerned). In the front part of the oral cavity the tip of the tongue always flicks during the utterance of the consonant *l* (in the words *pól* and *půl*). During *ú* in the word *půl* the throat cavity has the shape depicted in fig. 67. During *ú* and *í* there is a markedly similar movement of the root of the tongue. In no case of the pronunciation of spoken isolated vowels is the tip of the tongue raised towards the hard palate as was the case with the phonation of sung vowels by the same person.

In the articulatory movements in the given words the contact of the tip of the tongue with the hard palate during the consonant *l* is very clear. In cases of vowels situated in words are manifested articulatory formations typical for their pronunciation in isolation. During phonation there is very clearly visible muscular tension on the soft palate, and on the other hand during the short pauses between the individual examples it is seen relaxing.

Third series. Even during spoken vowels this test subject shows a special tongue motion during the phonation of front vowels. The tongue has a rounded shape for all vowels except *á* and *ó*. In general it is either thrust forward (for front vowels) or backwards (for back vowels). Fig. 68 shows schematically the position of the

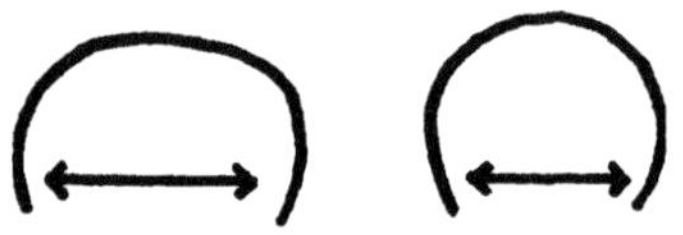

Fig. 68. Schematic diagram of the contraction of the tongue muscle in profile projection (3rd series – tip of the tongue to the right).

tongue. During the pronunciation of the words a marked horizontal contraction of the tongue muscle was visible in the profile projection. The tip of the tongue is in all cases except *á* and *ó* contracted on the floor of the oral cavity to the back. The vowel *é* sounds very closed. During *ó* the tip of the tongue is only on the floor of the oral cavity but tending forwards, not backwards (but it is however thrust further back than with *á*). Again the articulation of the consonant *l* is marked in the words *pól* and *půl*.

At an exposure rate of 24ps the affricate *c* and the stops *p* and *t* are inadequately recordable on the film shots for registering the articulatory movements during spoken sounds, owing to their short duration.

4. VOWELS SUNG WITH THE SAME INTENSITY AT DIFFERENT PITCHES[5]

4.1. *Low tones*

First series (g ♯ – 204 Hz). In all the vowels sung in the syllables *bí, bé, bá, bó, bú,* at 204 Hz there was not the same muscular tension as at 294 Hz. (fig. 69). Nor is the undulating motion of the tongue nearly so obvious as at the higher frequency. Of the given syllables sung at 204 Hz the tongue is most tensed during the syllable *bú* when during phonation its slight undulation is visible.

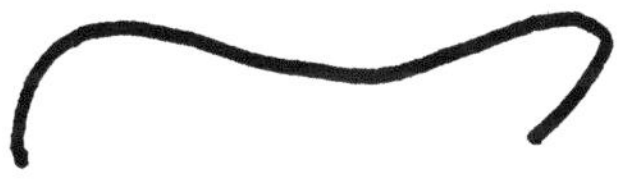

Fig. 69. Schematic diagram of the shape of the tongue during the pronunciation of *ú* sung at a frequency of 204 Hz (1st series – tip of the tongue to the right).

The motion of the tongue is such as is habitually described for the articulation of the vowels *í, é, á, ó, ú.* From the acoustic stand-point all the syllables are identifiable as *bí, bé, bá, bó, bú.* At a frequency of 204 Hz there is manifested a particular undulation of the tongue which does not occur on the other shots of the subject. The undulation precedes from the rear forwards. It is caused by the fact that the back of the tongue arches a fraction of a second earlier than the front.

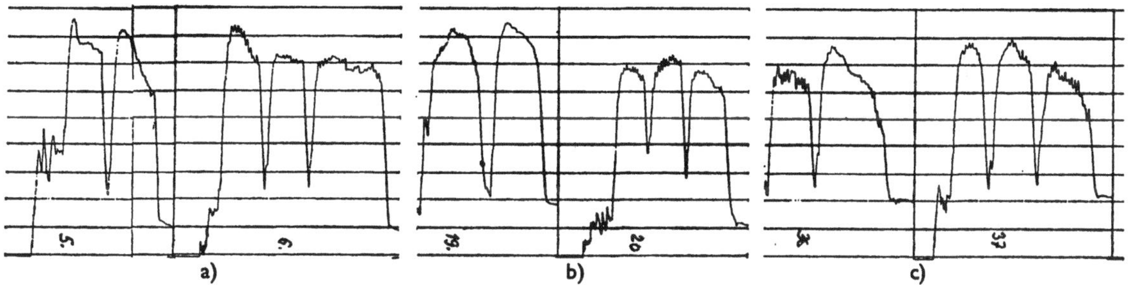

Fig. 70. Recording of the intensity of the syllables *bí, bé, bá, bó, bú,* (a) sung at a frequency of 204 Hz – 1st series, (b) sung at 184 Hz – 2nd series, (c) sung at 174 Hz – 3rd series.

[5] The shots of the first series (RJ) were realised at frequencies of 204, 294, 348, 408, and 367 Hz; the second series (RA) at frequencies of 184, 261, 306, 367 and 326 Hz, and the third series (JH) at frequencies of 232, 174, 204, 232 and 209 Hz. (With the third series the realisations were made on lower tones than intended, with 174 Hz instead of 348 Hz, 204 Hz instead of 408 Hz, 232 Hz instead of 464 Hz and 209 Hz instead of 418 Hz.) Intensity should be understood in the relative conception of the individual test subjects.

The designation of low tone, high tone and highest tone is relative in respect to the vocal range of the test subjects.

Second series ($f\sharp$ – 184 Hz). In all the vowels the tongue (not only its tip) is raised during the holding of the tone towards the hard palate. The tension of the tongue is very strong and so it is raised throughout its whole length. The tip of the tongue is not turned up vertically. The contour of the tongue shows the position typical for the individual vowels. The flattest is during *á*, the most rounded during *ó* and *ú* when it is drawn back. On the other hand during *í* and *é* it tends forwards.

Third series (f – 174 Hz). On a shot of the articulation of the syllable *bí* can be seen that the epiglottis inclines toward the root of the tongue and that a velopharyngeal closure is created. The tongue is arched upwards and has a rounded shape. At the root of the tongue is visible a strong muscular pull causing a movement forwards to the lower incisors. During the articulation of the syllable *bé* the arching of the tongue is significantly narrowed in comparison with the foregoing articulatory position. Although the arching is narrower, it is lower in relation to the hard palate than during the articulation of *bí*. This is shown schematically in fig. 71. During the syllables *bí*

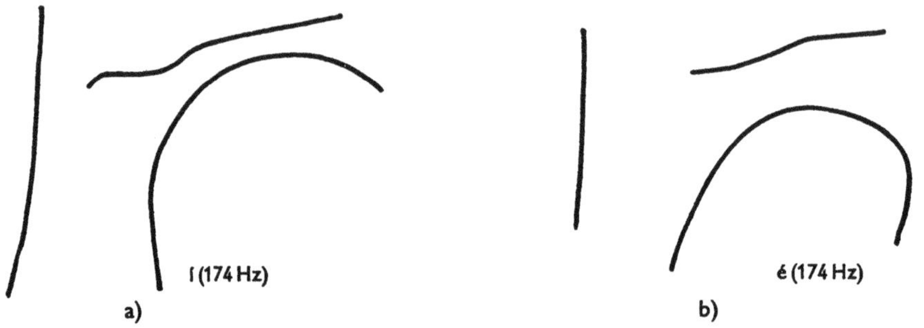

Fig. 71. Schematic representation of the different arching of the tongue (a) during *í* sung in the syllable *bí* (wider), and (b) during *é* sung in the syllable *bé* (narrower and lower).

and *bé* the contour of the rear wall of the soft palate and the uvula is roughly parallel with the contour of the rear wall of the throat. During the articulation of *bá*, *bó*, and *bú* the contour of the uvula inclines away from the rear wall of the throat. The upper part of the rear wall of the soft palate does not make the same contact with the rear wall of the throat; the area of contact is smaller and is only in the upper part.

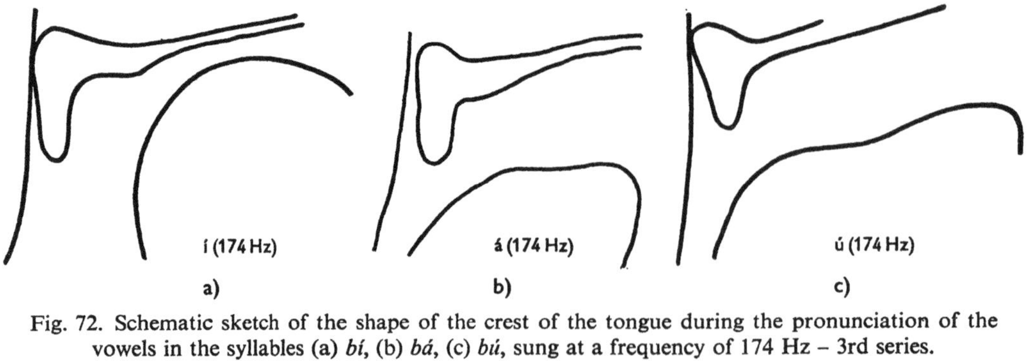

Fig. 72. Schematic sketch of the shape of the crest of the tongue during the pronunciation of the vowels in the syllables (a) *bí*, (b) *bá*, (c) *bú*, sung at a frequency of 174 Hz – 3rd series.

In so far as a velopharyngeal closure is realised it is in differing degrees, which is caused by the various relative positions of the rear wall of the soft palate and the rear wall of the throat and their varying muscular tension.

The shape of the crest of the tongue is roughly the same as at a frequency of 232 Hz. During the syllable *bú* the tongue is lowest, and its crest is markedly flexed. For schematic representation see fig. 72.

4.2. *Medium tones*

First series (d^1 – 294 Hz). When the syllable *bí* is sung there is a very marked right closure. With the syllable *bé* a narrow passage is visible between the rear wall of the throat and the soft palate; this passage is greater during the singing of the syllable *bá*. With the syllable *bó* the passage is again reduced though it is still greater than with *bé*. Instead of the last syllable *bú* was realised, and identified by ear, the syllable *bó*. If we compare the syllables *bí, bé, bá, bó* sung at a frequency of 294 Hz according to the relative position of the rear wall of the throat and the soft palate (from a tight closure up to a passage to the nasal cavity) we arrive at the order *bí, bó, bé, bá*.

The muscular tension of the soft palate during the articulation of the vowel is coordinated with that of the tongue. During singing at a frequency of 294 Hz the muscular tension of the tongue is strongest with the syllable *bí*, less with the syllable *bó* and least with the syllable *bá*.

For the test subject of the first series the undulating contour of the tongue during the articulation of sung vowels besides *í* is characteristic. During the articulation of the syllable *bé* a wavy movement of the tongue runs from the back forwards, while during the articulation of the other three syllables *bá, bó, bó* the wavy movement runs backwards from the front. When projected this wavy movement during the order *bé, bá, bó, bó* first gives the impression of pressure from the back forwards and presently from the front backwards. This movement is most marked in the second realisation of the syllable *bó*. The wavy movement of the tongue is further emphasised by the fact that between the phonation of the individual syllables there is muscular relaxation in the short pauses between the syllables.

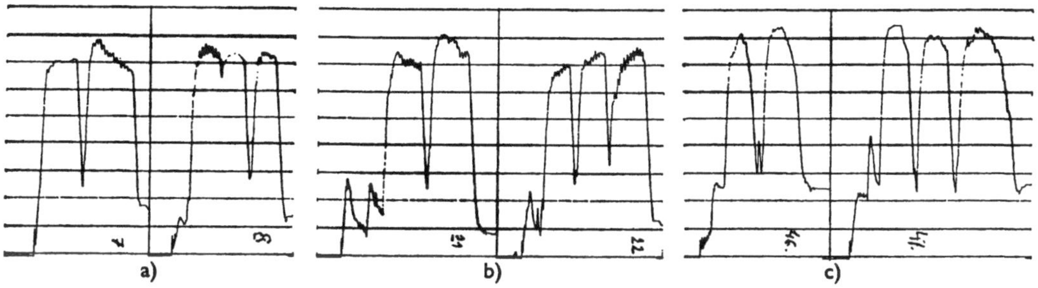

a) b) c)

Fig. 73. Recording of the intensity of the syllables *bí, bé, bá, bó, bú* sung at the frequencies (a) 294 Hz – 1st series, (b) 261 Hz – 2nd series, (c) 204 Hz – 3rd series.

Second series (c^1 – 261 Hz). During the articulation of the syllables *bí* and *bú* (syllables with the extreme vowels at each end of the scale) there are clear vibrations of the root of the tongue. Tension of the tongue is less than at a frequency of 184 Hz. With the syllables *bá, bó, bú* the tongue is raised during phonation. The overall tendency in the movement of the tongue muscle at this frequency (261 Hz) is: with *bí* forward and upward; with *bé*, compared with the preceding *bí*, further back and upward; with *bá* well back with the tip of the tongue starting in a low position but during phonation the whole area of the front part of the tongue moves upwards; with *bó* and *bú* also the front part of the tongue moves upward during phonation. In relative terms the tongue is least active during *é*. The rear part of the tongue at its summit is furthest from the soft palate during the articulation of the vowel *í* and closest during *ú*.

Third series (g ♯ – 204 Hz). During the articulation of the syllables *bí* and *bé* a

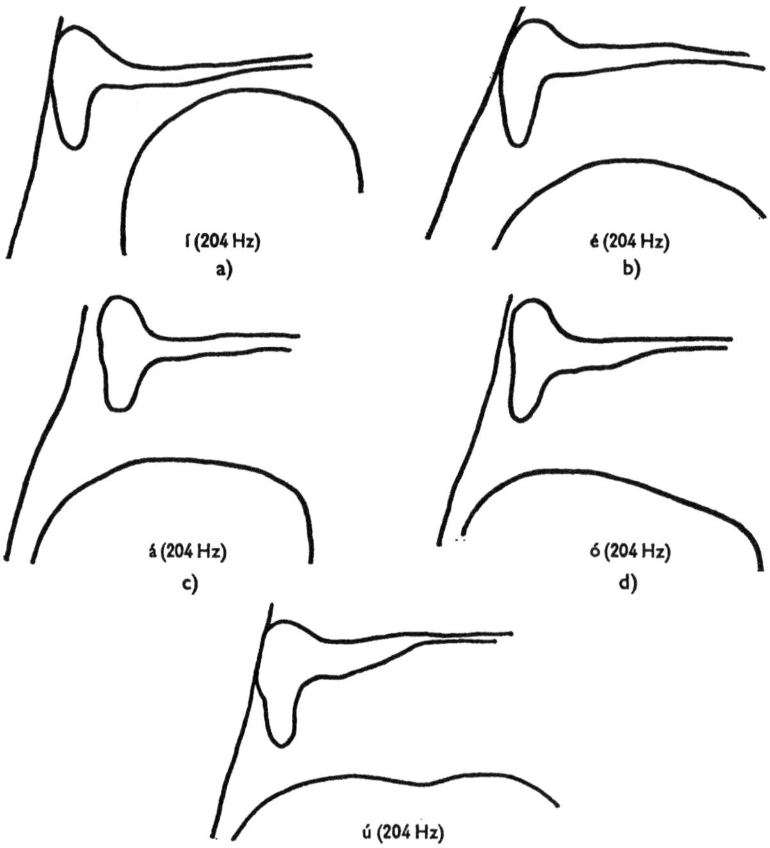

Fig. 74. Schematic illustration of the shape of the tongue during the pronunciation of the vowels in the syllables *bí, bé, bá, bó, bú* sung at a frequency of 204 Hz – 3rd series.

velopharyngeal closure is manifested when projected; during the articulation of *bá*, *bó* and *bú* a free passage to the nasal cavity is observable. The passage is narrowest with the syllable *bú*, widest with the syllable *bá*.

All in all there is no great muscular tonus during the singing of the syllables at 204 Hz. Tonus is however greater on the tongue than on the soft palate.

The shape of the tongue is shown schematically in fig. 74.

4.3. *Higher tones*

First series (f^1 – 348 Hz). The influence of a relatively high tone produces in test subject I a strong neutralisation of vowels. Instead of the desired syllables *bí* and *bé* we hear */h/é* and */h/é* with an unclear *é*. We identify the last of the vowels as *ó* and *ó* instead of the desired syllables *bó* and *bú*. Only the vowel *á* is clear.

Quite striking is the unusual shape of the tongue. During the articulation of the first two syllables it is arched upwards in its rear part. During the articulation of the remaining three syllables the tongue is not so upward arched; it is slightly curved and at the same time undulated. This curving may be ascribed to the great muscular effort of the person in singing at this pitch (348 Hz).

The jaw angle is markedly smaller in the first two syllables than in the other three.

The soft palate shows no great muscular tension. Nor in any one case does it form a velopharyngeal closure with the rear wall of the throat. During all five phonated sounds the narrow velopharyngeal passage remains at more or less the same width.

In the transition from the last phase of phonation to the phase without phonation can be clearly seen a phase of the first degree of muscular relaxation on the soft palate; the muscular relaxation does not take place all at once.

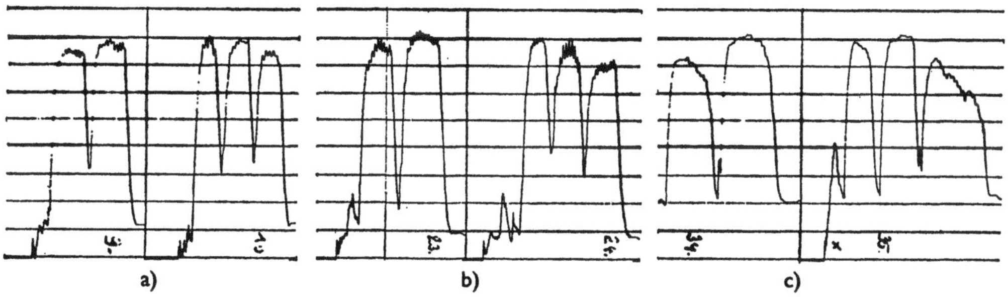

Fig. 75. Recording of the intensity of the syllables *bí, bé, bá, bó, bú* (a) sung at a frequency of 348 Hz – 1st series, (b) sung at a frequency of 306 Hz – 2nd series, (c) sung at a frequency of 232 Hz – 3rd series.

Second series (d $\sharp^1$ – 306 Hz). The velopharyngeal closure is strongest during the articulation of the syllable *bí*; during *bé* it is weakest. Even during *bú* there is relatively little tension on the soft palate. The contour shape of the crest of the tongue is similar to that during articulation at 261 Hz though the tongue has greater muscular tension. The tip of the tongue is more raised and in this way deviates from continuous line of the crest of the tongue.

Third series (b ♭ – 232 Hz). With the sung syllables *bá, bó* there is a narrow but clear velopharyngeal closure; with *bú* the closure is not secure and contact in the upper part of the rear wall of the soft palate is made with the rear wall of the throat. During the articulation of the syllables *bí* and *bé* a velopharyngeal closure of varying nature is realised. While during the articulation of the syllable *bí* the rear wall of the

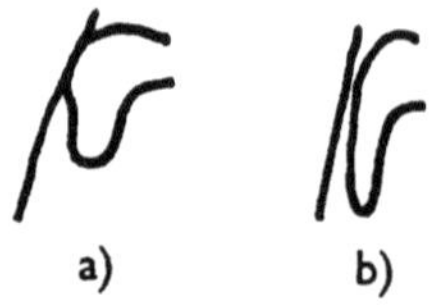

Fig. 76. Schematic illustration of the different shape of the soft palate in relation to the rear wall of the throat, (a) during the vowel *í* in the sung syllable *bí*, (b) during the vowel *é* in the sung syllable *bé* (both at a frequency of 232 Hz – 3rd series).

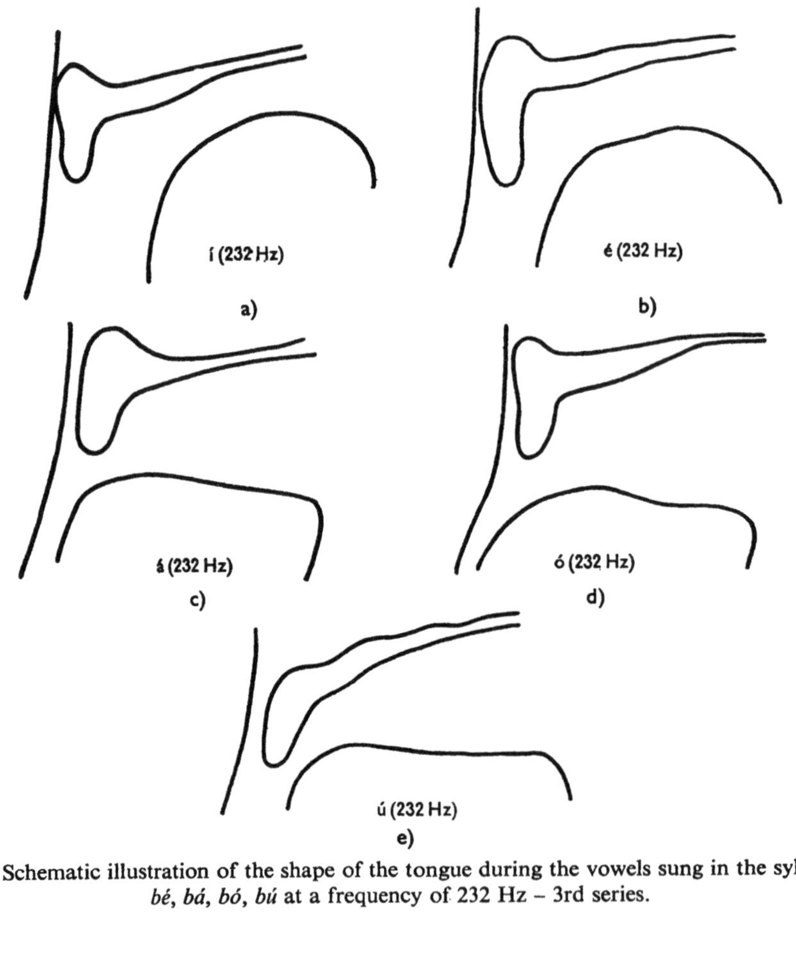

Fig. 77. Schematic illustration of the shape of the tongue during the vowels sung in the syllables *bí, bé, bá, bó, bú* at a frequency of 232 Hz – 3rd series.

soft palate is curved and makes contact with the rear wall of the throat, with *bé* the soft palate and the uvula are pulled further down so that the contact is markedly interrupted. (fig. 76.)

During the articulation of the syllable *bí* the tongue has a rounded shape; with *bé* it changes to parabolic. During *bá* it is flattened in the middle of the crest with quite steep side walls formed by the tip of the tongue and the upper part of its root. The level of the crest of the tongue during the following *bó* tends obliquely downwards towards the lower incisors. During the articulatory phase of the syllable *bú* there is a marked curving of the tongue in the middle of the crest from which comes the undulation. The tip of the tongue and the rear part of the crest are almost at the same level. The schematic presentation of this is in fig. 77.

4.4. *The highest tones*

First series (g $\sharp^1$ – 408 Hz). In no case is there a velopharyngeal closure. Against the desired syllables *bí, bé, bá, bó, bú*, the acoustic impression of the sung syllables is */h/é, /h/é, /h/á, bó, bó*. The widest gap between rear wall of the throat and the soft palate is with the syllable *bó*. The soft palate is less tensed than at a frequency of 348 Hz. It is not very much arched away from the level which it forms with the hard palate. The velopharyngeal gap at this frequency 408 Hz is the widest in comparison with the three lower frequencies of the first series. During the first two syllables */h/é* and */h/é* the soft palate has greater muscular tension than during the other three – */h/á, bó, bó*. It is arched though not very high in relation to the level of the hard palate. In its arched part it approaches the rear wall of the throat. In the remaining three syllables the soft palate is not arched. Its upper contour is even lowered in relation to the level of the hard palate, particularly during the final *ó*. In this case however we must also take into account the potential influence of the transition to the position without phonation.

There is clearly visible on the tongue strong muscular tension. During the first syllables there is strong pressure of the tongue from the back forwards and in the

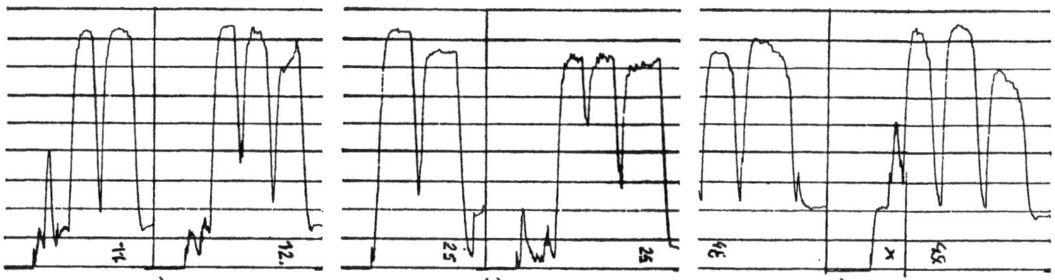

Fig. 78. Recording of the intensity of the syllables *bí, bé, bá, bó, bú*, (a) sung at a frequency of 408 Hz – 1st series, (b) sung at a frequency of 367 Hz – 2nd series, (c) sung at a frequency of 232 Hz – 3rd series.

others from the front backwards. In the first two syllables the tongue is arched in the front part; in the other three in the back part. There is greater muscular tension in the tongue than in the soft palate.

In the first series the raising of the frequency has the result of widening the velopharyngeal gap, reducing the muscular tension in the soft palate, lowering the upward arching of the upper part of the soft palate in relation to the level of the hard palate, but increasing the muscular tension of the tongue. From the point of view of the auditory impression the increase in frequency produces marked neutralisation of the vowels *í* and *ú*; *í* is identified as *é*, and *ú* as *ó*. This means that at higher frequencies for the test subject of the first series the pronunciation of extreme vowels, i.e. the vowels requiring strong muscular tension, creates a difficulty. In spite of quite a wide velopharyngeal passage the vowels have no nasal colouring.

Second series (f $\sharp^1$ – 367 Hz). Muscular tension is very strong. It is particularly clear on the tongue. Whereas at the three lower frequencies with the test subject of the second series the tonus of the tongue was manifested in that during the phonation of the individual vowels the tongue was raised in the greater part of its mass upwards towards the hard palate. At a frequency of 367 Hz, however, the tension of the tongue is shown by a raising upwards of the tip towards the hard palate (except for the articulatory position during the phonation of the vowel *í* where the tip of the tongue remains drawn down, though above the upper incisors).

During the pronunciation of the syllables *bí* and *bé* the soft palate is highest and has very strong muscular tension. During the syllable *bá* a passage to the nasal cavity is manifested. Quite striking is the lesser degree of arching of the soft palate during the back vowels than during the front vowels, which is naturally demonstrated also by the obtuseness and acuteness of the angle between the planes of the hard and soft palates. Also very marked is the activity of the rear wall of the throat, i.e. its arching and approach to the rear wall of the soft palate.

Third series (b♭ – 232 Hz). This realisation was repeated. In the sung syllable *bí* appears a velopharyngeal closure; with *bé* there is a narrow passage between the rear wall of the throat and the soft palate. The syllables *bá* and *bó* do not produce the velopharyngeal closure, and during the singing of the syllable *bú* the soft palate makes a weak contact with the rear wall of the throat.

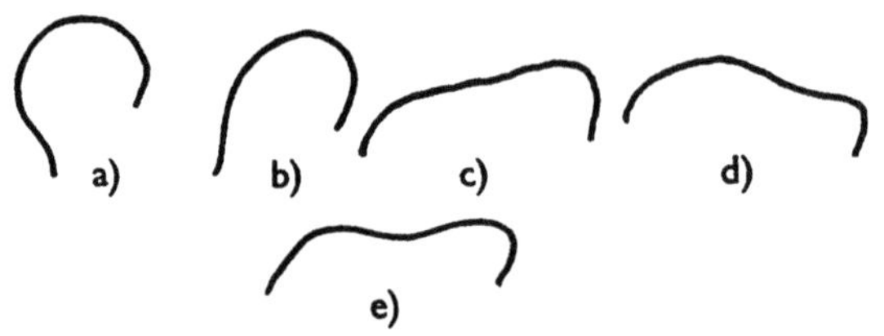

Fig. 79. Schematic illustration of the shape of the tongue during the vowels sung (a) in the syllable *bí*, (b) in the syllable *bé*, (c) in the syllable *bá*, (d) in the syllable *bó*, (e) in the syllable *bú* (frequency 232 Hz – 3rd series).

During *bí* the tongue has a rounded shape. During *bé* the profile of the tongue is drawn out. During the articulation of the syllable *bá* the crest of the tongue shows very slight undulation. This undulation takes place in grades – with the syllable *bó* it is quite strong and with *bú* it is most discernible. At the same time there is a change in the general trend of the tongue. (fig. 79).

5. CHANGES IN THE INTENSITY OF THE TONE

5.1. *Pianissimo*

First series (f $\sharp^1$ / 367 Hz). In all syllables there is a marked wide velopharyngeal gap. The general muscular tension is not particularly strong. There is no case of a velopharyngeal closure. With the syllable *bí* the soft palate is highest (greatest tension) and with the syllable *bá* is lowest (least tension).

Second series (e^1 – 326 Hz). The tonus of the soft palate is very great. The soft palate touches the rear wall of the throat during *bí*; in the other syllables the tonus is less and there is no such contact. During *í* the tongue is highest. Of great interest is the articulatory movement which comes from the root of the tongue. When sung vowels are held the tongue has, at the commencement of the phonation of the syllables *bá, bó, bú*, a rounded shape, during the phonation the tip of the tongue lifts upwards toward the hard palate. It really forms a barrier to the phonational current, which does not agree with earlier data about the free oral cavity with the spoken vowels. Not even the acoustic impression is affected by this movement of the tongue during the articulation (no detectable noises are produced). The given vowels *á, ó,* and *ú* are safely identified.

On the film are very clearly visible the well-known differences in the capacity of the throat and oral cavities during the front vowels (*í, é*) as against the capacity of the same cavities during the back vowels (*ó* and *ú*). In the first case the throat cavity is large and the oral cavity small; in the second the reverse is true.

Third series (a $\flat$ – 209 Hz). The test subject sings only the vowels. Before the vowels *í* and *á* one can clearly detect the preparation of the speech organs for the phonation. During *ó* the tongue has an unusual shape. As against the characteristic motion of the tongue during *ó*, the crest of the tongue is flat and slightly undulated. During *é* however the tongue has a rounded shape (whereas normally with this vowel

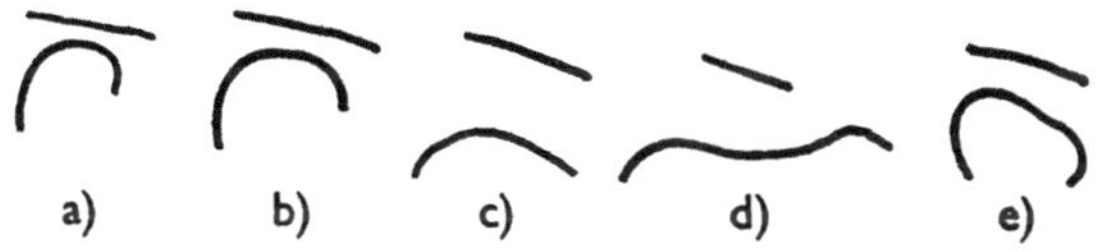

Fig. 80. Schematic illustration of the shape of the tongue during the sung vowels (a) *bí*, (b) *bé*, (c) *bá*, (d) *bó*, (e) *bú* (frequency 418 Hz – 3rd series – lips to the right).

the crest of the tongue is drawn out). Though muscular tonus is visible on the soft palate, this is not noticeably great. (fig. 80). During the articulation of the vowels the velopharyngeal closure is visible; it is least with *á*. All the vowels are very easily identifiable by ear.

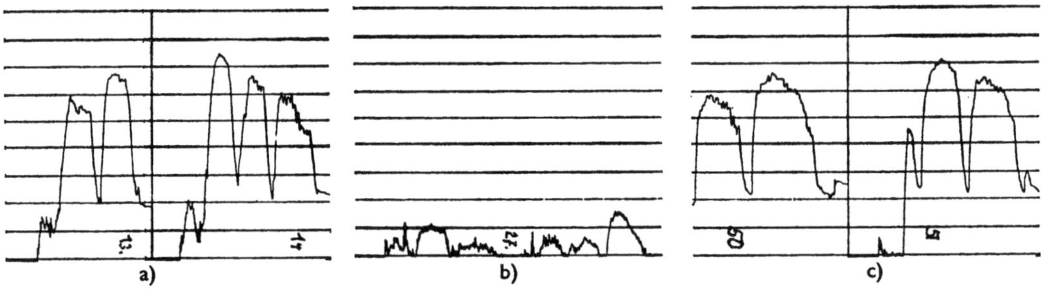

Fig. 81. Recording of the intensity of the syllables *bí, bé, bá, bó, bú* (a) sung at a frequency of 367 Hz – 1st series, (b) sung at a frequency of 326 Hz – 2nd series, (c) sung at a frequency of 418 Hz – 3rd series (pianissimo).

5.2. *Mezzoforte*

First series (f $\sharp^1$ – 367 Hz). With all the sung vowels there is a wide velopharyngeal gap. The main direction of movement of the tongue is with the first two vowels forwards and upwards, and in the three last vowels backwards and upwards. The overall impression from the articulatory position reminds one rather of the position with pianissimo than with fortissimo. Muscular tension is least (in comparison with pianissimo and fortissimo). In the test subject of the first series the greatest muscular tension is with fortissimo.

The upper contour of the soft palate is raised and curved in comparison with the level of the hard palate. Tension on the soft palate is not particularly marked and is manifested merely by a raising of the soft palate, though not at all by its approaching the rear wall of the throat. The tension of the soft palate is also clearly manifested by its being shortened in the middle part.

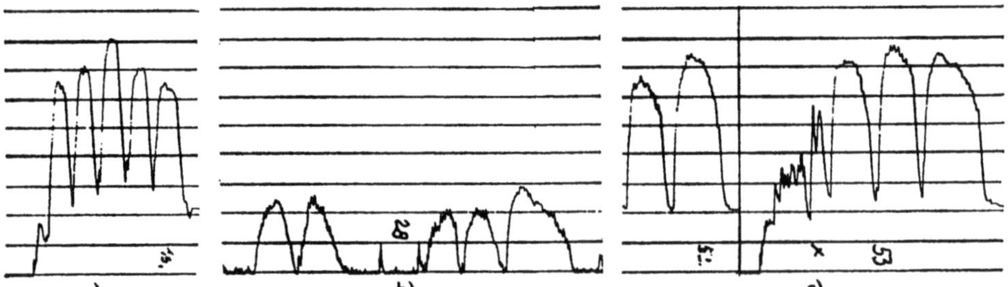

Fig. 82. Recording of the intensity of the syllables *bí, bé, bá, bó, bú* (a) sung at a frequency of 367 Hz – 1st series, (b) at a frequency of 326 Hz – 2nd series, (c) at a frequency of 209 Hz – 3rd series (mezzoforte).

Second series (e^1 – 326 Hz). The soft palate shows marked muscular tonus which however is less than with pianissimo. The whole mass of the tongue goes upwards /*bí*/, forwards /*bé*/ and backwards /*bá, bó, bú*/. At the beginning of the phonation the tip of the tongue is always down, but during the course of the phonation rises upwards. The greatest muscular tonus of the soft palate is during *í* and *é*, and it is noticeably less in the other vowels. All the vowels are easily identifiable.

Third series (a ♭ – 209 Hz). Only a hint of the consonant *b* is heard at the beginning of the syllable. On the whole there is less muscular tonus than at pianissimo in the same person. In the articulation of the vowel *ú* the crest of the tongue has a different shape than when *ú* is sung pianissimo.

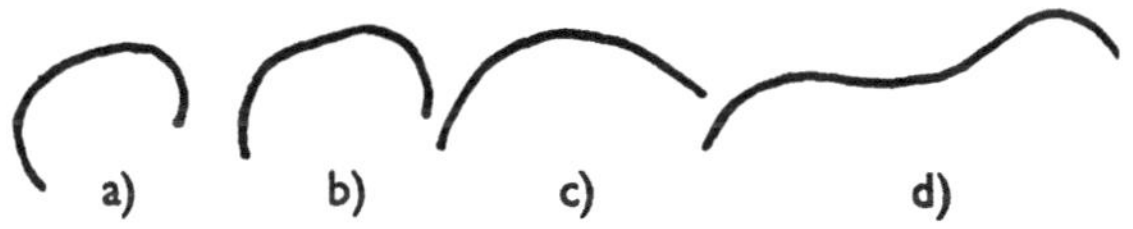

Fig. 83. Schematic illustration of the shape of the tongue in the syllables (a) *bí*, (b) *bé*, (c) *bá*, (d) *bó*. 3rd series – 209 Hz.

The remaining vowels preserve the character of the tongue contour much the same as during pianissimo (fig. 83). Very striking is the great difference in the mode of articulation of the test subjects of series two and three.

5.3. *Fortissimo*

First series (f $\sharp^1$ – 367 Hz). During sung *í* there is a velopharyngeal closure; in the remaining vowels there is not. Instead of the vowel *ú* is clearly identified *ó*. (The test subject of the first series has greatest difficulty in maintaining the pronunciation of the vowel *ú*). Instead of the initial consonant *b* in the first two syllables /*bí, bé*/ an unclear *h* is realised. The least muscular tension of the soft palate is visible in the utterance of the last *ó;* the strongest is with *í*. This tension is further manifested in a raising of the soft palate. During *í* the soft palate is highest, with *é* it is lower and with the remaining vowels it gets lower and lower until with the final *ó* it is at its lowest. The crest of the tongue during the first two vowels tends forwards and upwards and in the last three backwards and upwards. The muscular tension of the tongue is greater than that of the soft palate.

Generally the test subject of the first series manifests, inter al., greater muscular tension of the tongue and of the soft palate during fortissimo. The tension of the soft palate takes place by contraction in a horizontal direction, and by its being raised, though not by any approach to the rear wall of the throat. This type of muscular tension of the soft palate is specific to the test subject of the first series, in the same way as in this person is always manifested greater tension on the tongue than on the soft palate.

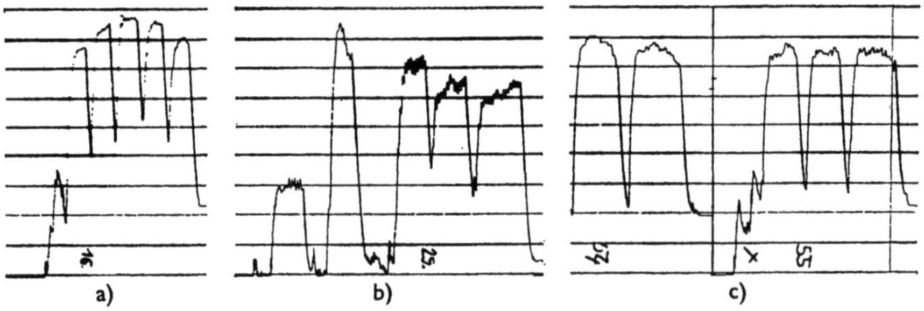

Fig. 84. Recording of the intensity of the syllables *bí, bé, bá, bó, bú,* (a) sung at a frequency of 367 Hz – 1st series, (b) sung at a frequency of 326 Hz – 2nd series, (c) sung at a frequency of 209 Hz – 3rd series (fortissimo).

Second series (e^1 – 326 Hz). With all five vowels there is a velopharyngeal closure. The tip of the tongue rises in the course of the phonation vertically upwards towards the hard palate with the syllables *bé, bá, bó, bú* (the shot of the syllable *bí* does not catch the tip of the tongue). The muscular tonus of the soft palate and the tongue is very strong. The tongue is most rounded during the production of *bó*.

Third series (a ♭ – 209 Hz). The acoustic impression of the sung syllables is */p/bí/*, *bé, bá, bó, bó*. The contour of the tongue has an unusual shape. With *í* the tongue is rounded. In comparison with its motion with the other vowels it is at its closest (i.e. highest) to the hard palate. During the syllable *bé* the tongue is lower and its shape is again almost round. During *á* and the first *ó* the outline of the tongue is flattened and in the case of the last *ó* the tongue is arched only in its rear part; the crest and the tip of the tongue incline obliquely towards the lower incisors. The soft palate has greatest muscular tonus during *í;* it is pressed up against the rear wall of the throat. During the production of the last vowel a weak transition from *u* to *o* is heard, i.e. *b*^{ú}*ó;* from the commencement of this phonation a slight undulation of the tongue is visible on the X-ray photograph.[6]

6. CONTINUOUS SUNG SCALE

First series. The scale is sung on a neutral vowel. The soft palate arches upwards with the rise in tone; when the highest tone is sustained the soft palate remains in the upper position. The cineradiographic shot records the scale being sung upwards. The crest of the tongue gradually arches slightly up in accordance as the tone is higher. It seems however that this movement is merely an accompaniment to the movement

[6] This shot is a proof of how very important is the exact synchrony of the sound recording and the cineradiographic recording. The change of the articulatory formation (not however every change) can be followed by an acoustic effect. On the other hand if when listening to the sound recording we detect a change in the timbre of the vowel we may be sure that we shall find the corresponding change on the film record of the movement of the speech-organs.

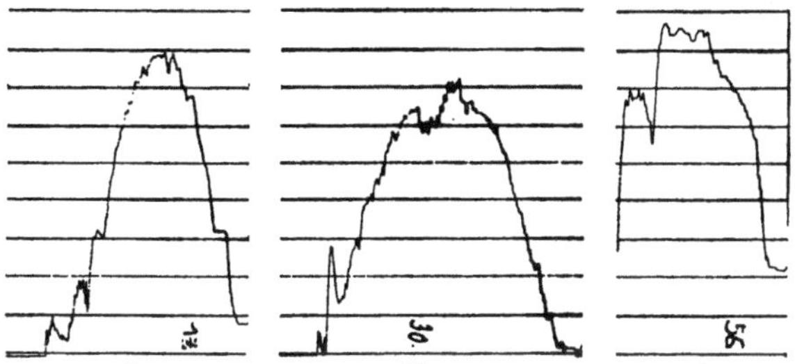

Fig. 85. Recording of the intensity of the continuous sung scale, (a) 1st series, (b) 2nd series, (c) 3rd series.

of the lower jaw which closes up slightly with the rising of the tone. At the highest sustained tone the jaw closes up markedly.

Second series. The scale is sung to the syllable *la* with *á* sustained. The acoustic impression is rather of a mixed vowel /ə/ than of pure *á*. At the end of the continuous scale there is again a clearly visible movement of the tip of the tongue towards the hard palate with the consonant *l;* that is to say the syllable *la* appears again, and in this case is more clearly identifiable as *la* than at the beginning.

This shot demonstrates that with sung vowels the articulatory motion of the tongue often has the tip upward. The position of the tongue as recorded on the sketch is maintained through the whole phonation of the scale sung up and down. On the shot it is visible how the tongue jumps up to the hard palate and touches it during the production of the consonant *l.*

At the highest tones there is a very clearly visible movement of the soft palate which is manifested in its moving away from the rear wall of the throat and then moving back again consequently causing the realisation of a velopharyngeal closure.

Third series. On the X-ray shots recording the continuous scale sung on the syllable *né* with *é* sustained the preparation for the phonation is very clearly visible, especially on the soft palate. The soft palate already has tonus during this preparation, it is raised, but its upper face is not arched upwards. The tonus is clear also on the rear part of the tongue during this preparatory phase.

At the beginning of the phonation the soft palate is abruptly lifted. It keeps this position during the phonation of the first tone sustained on *né.* With the next tone the soft palate rises still more (which gives the impression of 'confirming' the articulatory position) and presses itself to the rear wall of the throat. In this way the velopharyngeal closure is made. It remains in this position through the other tones sung on *é.* At the first held tone no great degree of muscular tension is visible on the tongue; at the next tone on the scale its tension increases markedly, the jaw angle is enlarged, and the tip of the tongue is contracted behind the lower incisors. As the tone rises so the tension on the tongue increases, which is manifested also by an undulation of the contour of its crest.

7. SUPPLEMENT TO THE ANALYSES OF THE SHOTS OF THE CONTINUOUS SUNG SCALE

7.1. *Photograph centred on the area of the uvula*

Second series. The scale is sung on a mixed vowel /ə/ in spite of the fact that the test subject was supposed to be singing *la*. The most interesting point on this shot is the alternating approaching and distancing of the soft palate and the rear wall of the throat. This movement of the soft palate occurs only when the scale is sung upwards (the soft palate vibrates five times); when the scale is sung downwards, there is no such movement. During these movements of the soft palate towards the rear wall of the throat as described, the soft palate is strongly tensed which is shown by the way it is greatly arched upwards even when moving away from the rear wall of the throat. The tongue is curved throughout the whole period of phonation.

Third series (sung on the syllable *né/é/*). The preparation for phonation is seen particularly in the muscular tension of the soft palate. With the initial held tone on *né* the soft palate rises abruptly. It is not yet however at its maximum height (within the scope of the articulatory movement of this shot). This it reaches at the second tone on the scale and remains there for almost the whole period of phonation of the other tones on the scale. During the three or two last tones (the scale is sung continuously so it is difficult to speak of the individual tones) a lessening of the muscular tension of the soft palate sets in, which allows us to conclude a velopharyngeal passage.

7.2. *Shot from the lips over the tongue and soft palate to the upper part of the larynx*

Second series. A tone sustained on *é* with uncertain consonant at the beginning is sung though it sounds rather more like a mixed vowel. The tongue is not curved and the tip has an upward trend. Throughout the duration of phonation the soft palate forms a velopharyngeal closure with the rear wall of the throat. A slight flicker of the tongue, i.e. its contact with the alveolae, appears right at the beginning of the phonation of this shot. Acoustically it most resembles *n*. The root of the tongue vibrates slightly towards the rear wall of the throat.

Third series. The scale is sung to *né*. With the initial *n* there is clear contact of the tongue with the alveolae. The tip of the tongue is not on the floor of the oral cavity but tends forwards to the cutting edge of the lower incisors. The crest of the tongue is arched towards the hard palate. There is no marked change in the tonus of the tongue and the soft palate during the phonation in the course of the scale. The tonus of the soft palate is not very great (it makes a light closure with the wall of the throat). As against the usual position during the vowel *é* there appears here a relatively large distance of the crest of the tongue from the hard palate. Very clear is the movement of the root of the tongue in the horizontal plane. The way it approaches and withdraws from the rear wall of the throat appears particularly clearly.

V

CONCLUSIONS

1. THE ARTICULATION OF THE SUNG, SPOKEN AND WHISPERED CZECH VOWELS *í, é, á, ó, ú*

From the comparison of the results of the mentioned analyses showing the articulatory phases and movements of the speech-organs during the articulation of long Czech vowels sung, spoken and whispered by the same person it is seen that the speech organs maintain their basic characteristic motion for the given vowel whether it is sung, spoken or whispered.[1]

It is almost a rule that the oral cavity increases progressively from whispered, through spoken, to sung vowels, as long as they are realized the middle register of the test subject. The oral cavity is freed by the tongue's overall contraction downwards to the floor of the cavity, while maintaining the typical shape for the given vowel. In such a case neither the jaw angle nor the labial gap show any great change as a rule.[2]

This way of freeing the oral cavity was discovered in all the test subjects in the realization of the vowels *í* and *ú* for which the smallest jaw angle is characteristic.[3]

In other cases an enlarging of the oral cavity is achieved by a combination of a change in the jaw angle and the position of the tongue (again keeping the characteristic shape for the given vowel). In this case however we could not discover a regular enlarging of the oral cavity in the direction whispering-speaking-singing; in the realization of the vowels by the individual test subjects there appeared considerably different methods. Because the production of *é*, *á* and *ó* is a more complex phenom-

[1] In this comparison we take account of the vowel as sung mezzoforte at the mean pitch of the vocal range of the test subject. The articulatory movements of the speech-organs in the individual subjects show individual forms (variations); in spite of this however even with these realisations (sometimes individual) such acoustic results are achieved as are identified as the same vowel.

According to Chlumský (*Česká kvantita, melodie a přízvuk*, Praha 1928, pp. 55-6) the length of short vowels was measured in centiseconds: for *i*, 5.25-5.5; for *e*, 9; for *a*, 10.5-12; for *o*, 8.5-9; for *u*, 6. Values measured for the long vowels were, in centiseconds: for *í*, 20.25-20.5; for *é*, 22-22.5; for *á*, 24-25.5; for *ó*, 21.5-22.5; for *ú*, 15.5-17.25. (B. Hála, *Uvedení do fonetiky češtiny na obecně fonetickém základě*, Praha 1962, p. 186.)

[2] With the labial aperture remaining at the same width we observed differences in the form of protruded lips particularly with the rounded vowels.

[3] Cf. e.g. the sketch of the articulatory formation of the speech-organs during *í* – 323 Z – fig. 8, 261 M – fig. 12, 313 Š – fig. 16 in their realisation by test subject RJ, sketches 212 Z – fig. 9, 183 M – fig. 13, 192 Š – fig. 17 of test subject RV etc.

enon than the previous case concerning *í* and *ú*, we shall present here its realization. With the vowel *é* the size of the jaw angle shows marked fluctuation. The tongue is not lowered passively with the lowering of the bottom jaw, but simultaneously changed its position in the oral cavity (within the framework of the characteristic shape for *é*).

With the vowel *á* there are marked individual realizations in the different test subjects. While with test subjects RV, MN, and LŠ it was not possible to discover any very great increase in the jaw angle as the size of the oral cavity was sufficiently altered by the tongue motion, in test subject RJ there was a twofold increase in the jaw angle. Simultaneously with the increase of the jaw angle there was a change in the shape of the tongue. During spoken and whispered *á* the tongue was mildly arched towards the hard palate and the alveolae; but when *á* was sung it was slightly undulated, lowered overall and partially thrust back. The tip was turned up.

Equally only with test subject RJ was there found a fundamental change in the jaw angle in the realization of the vowel *ó* when sung. The change was similar to that with *á*. All the test subjects showed a change in the jaw angle in the realization of *ó* sung at different pitches.[4]

On the other hand the enlargement of the oral cavity is not so regular with a change in intensity. If we start for example from a medium intensity /mf/ of the vowel sung at e^1 (sketch 335 – fig. 42) the jaw angle remains the same with *ó* sung forte at e^1 (sketch 222 – fig. 45), the crest of the tongue lowers and the tonus of the soft palate and the uvula drops somewhat. With pianissimo *ó* sung at a^1 (sketch 218 – fig. 43) the jaw angle is somewhat reduced and the crest of the tongue also drops, though not of course so much as with forte.

From the material it follows that any specific formation of the front part of the oral cavity is not strictly relevant for the auditive perception or identification of the vowels. The formation of the cavity is governed by the movement of the tongue, which in profile is seen in its various outlines (e.g. in its undulation). Nor is the size of the jaw angle strictly relevant. Of importance however is the overall relation between the capacity of the oral cavity and that of the throat. For example during *í* there is a noticeably large throat cavity and on the contrary a very small and narrow oral cavity.[5]

In two test subjects the course of the articulation with the increase of tone was quite different.[6] It is necessary to bear in view the relativity of tonal pitch in individual test subjects. Although in each case it is a matter of a different tone increase, the jaw angle has always an almost twofold increase at the higher tone, as against the angel

[4] We took the greater number of shots of the articulatory organs with a change in pitch during the vowel *ó* which was chosen for the experiments for the reason that none of the test subjects considered its pronunciation during singing to be difficult.

[5] Cf. e.g. G. Fant, Formants and cavities. *Proceedings of the V. International Congress of Phonetic Sciences Münster 1964*, Hague 1968.

[6] For example R. Curry was interested in similar problem as early as 1938 in "The Physiology of the Contralto Voice", *ANPE* XIV (1938) 73-79.

at a tone at the mean pitch of the vocal range of the same person. On sketch 354 (fig. 40) is illustrated the articulation of *ó* sung at a tonal pitch of g^2 mf; sketch 340 (fig. 39) at e^2 and sketch 352 (fig. 41) at a^2 mf. When singing *ó* at a higher tone this test subject shows a very marked increase in the front part of the oral cavity by opening the jaws. The tongue follows the drop of the lower jaw and with the greater jaw angle the rear part of the tongue crest and the root of the tongue are thrust back to the rear wall of the throat, at which however the passage to the throat cavity remains essentially the same. On the other hand the soft palate has greater tension in all three cases. In two cases it closes the passage to the nasal cavity, and in the other a hair-breadth gap remains free. At higher tones the soft palate is however relaxed, in two cases so much so that the passage to the nasal cavity remains wide open. This shape of the soft palate is in strong contrast to its form with *ó* sung at c^2.[7]

With test subject RV the changes in the articulatory movement of the speech-organs with changes in pitch are not so marked. With *ó* sung at a^1 tonal pitches the jaw angle remains much the same (sketches 209, 218, 222 – fig. 44, 43, 45), only the tongue with a rise in pitch is raised, quite curved, and has the tip directed towards the alveolae and reaching the middle of the labial gap. With a raising of the tone to a^2 the jaw angle is slightly enlarged (sketch 333 – fig. 47), though the tongue is bent in such a way that the tip is raised and directed upwards and backwards the hard palate. Overall the tongue is lowered in accordance with the drop of the lower jaw. The soft palate shows an increase in its muscular tension as the tone goes higher so that with a^2 in a rounded shape it closes very firmly the passage to the nasal cavity, and it is raised well above the level of the hard palate. In one and the same test subject the articulatory shape of the speech-organs remains the same on the pair of shots of *ó* sung at c^1 and c^2, only that the tonus of the uvula and the soft palate is greater at the higher tone. In both cases however the passage to the nasal cavity is free.

When the vowels are sung at a relatively high tone we find in one of the test subjects so-called neutralisation of the vowels *í* and *é*. Instead of the desired syllables *bí* and *bé*, an indefinite long vowel with aspiration is heard; this combination sounds most like the syllables *hé* and *hé*.

2. THE CHANGE OF TONAL PITCH AND THE COLOURING OF THE VOWELS

Studies in this domain have already been carried out for example by Hermann,[8] Kaňka,[9] and Hála.[10] Recently the relation of tonal pitch and vocalic colouring has been the concern of, for example, R. Husson.[11]

[7] Cf. the speech-organs on sketches 354 and 352 (fig. 40, 41) as against sketch 342 (fig. 38).

[8] "Neue Beiträge zur Lehre von den Vokalen und ihrer Entstehung", 1911.

[9] *Podmínky umělých samohláskových zvuků* (Conditions of Artificial Vowel Sounds), 1927; according to him *ú* sung soprano at f ♯² sounds as *u* > *o*, and *a* as *a* > *e*. And it is impossible to sing pure *u* at f ♯².

[10] *Akustická podstata samohlásek*, 1941.

[11] "Die Höhe der Stimme ist völlig unabhängig von ihrer Intensität und ihrem Timbre, denn diese

In test subject MN (soprano) we discovered similarly to Hála at what maximum pitch it is still possible to identify safely the character of vowels. The highest tone which the test subject was capable of singing was a^2 (she is a trained professional singer). Hála for an untrained female soprano also gives a^2. However at this pitch the subject MN was able without effort to produce only a neutral sound and none of the Czech vowels was clear. For instance in the singing of the vowel *í* on tones from a^1 and up, *í* changed its vocalic quality at f^2, i.e. at the point where the register is, and ceased to be audible as *í*. Hála gives from d^2 a light colouring towards *é*, and from f^2 a greater colouring towards *é*. From g^2 the vowel ceased to be clear. With the same test subject we found that the highest tone at which vowels can be safely identified is e^2 for *í*, *é*, *á*, *ó*, and for *ú* it is c^2 if the same mean loudness is maintained. Hála gives for *í*, *é* and *ó* the note c^2, for *á* e^2, and a^1 for *ú*. He closes with this summary of the information:

"The ability to form vowels at all continues up to the note g^2; from this note onwards all the vowels changed into a sound of indefinite complexion. The vowels *ú* and *ó* lose their complexion immediately the note rises above its characteristic (i.e. with *ú* at a^1, with *ó* at e^2); á remains unchanged up to f^2; it keeps its complexion the longest of all the vowels, *é* and *í* lose their complexion as from d^2, i.e. as soon as the fundamental frequency is higher than the lower resonance of these vowels." (Op. cit. above.)

Höhe hängt nur von der Frequenz der Rekurrensimpulse ab, ist also ein rein neurologischer Akt. Hingegen sind die INTENSITÄT und das GLOTTISCHE TIMBRE eng aneinander gebunden, da beide von den gleichen Faktoren abhängen: dem subglottischen Druck und dem Tonus des Glottis-Sphinkters. Die Ausbreitung in dem pharyngo-bukkalen Rohr ändert dann sekundär das anfängliche glottische Timbre und die anfängliche Intensität, wie wir später sehen werden, aber sie würde in keinem Falle die ausgesandte Frequenz ändern können." "Der gegenwärtige Stand der physiologischen Phonetik", *Phonetica* 4 (1959) 1-32.

According to Husson there are three basic configurations of the acoustic channel with two or three cavities: type 1 (two glottal cavities and the oral cavity) gives a clear *a*; type 2 (larynx and mouth) gives, depending on the bucolabial degree of opening, vocalities of a^0, open *o*, closed *o* and *u*; type three (larynx and two oral cavities) gives vocalities of open *ö*, closed *ö* and *ü*, if the tongue is drawn back, and vocalities of open *ä*, closed *e* and *i*, if the tongue is thrust forward. The bucolabial degree of opening completes the differentiation. Husson examined the development of Hellwag's 10 basic vocalities and came to the following conclusions: "Die 'Deckung des Tones' trifft man im ersten Register um 300 Hz an: Die 'offenen' Vokale können nicht mehr hervorgebracht werden. Um 400-450 Hz geht man in das zweite Register über, und die vier 'offenen' Vokale erscheinen wieder. Um 600 Hz zeigt sich die 'Deckung des Tones' im zweiten Register, und die 'offenen' Vokale verschwinden erneut. Darüber hinaus werden die Vokale '*o*' und '*u*' weniger deutlich sein, da ihr zu tiefer bukkaler Formant nicht mehr in ihrem Kehlkopfklang auftritt. Im Oberteil dieses Registers werden nur noch '*i*', '*e*', '*ö*' und '*ü*' deutlich hervorgebracht. Gegen 900-1000 Hz tritt das dritte Register /wenn es existiert/ in Erscheinung, und die Vokale beschränken sich grosso modo nur noch auf '*i*' und '*e*'. Über 1500 Hz, im vierten Register, kann nur noch der Vokal '*i*' als einziger hervorgebracht werden." (Op. cit.)

Husson goes on to state that Hellwag's triangle is modified if we go up the tonal scale, that in principle it is narrowed and forms above the base a body which he has called "allgemeine Vokalpyramide".

According to Strouhal[12] most frequent deformation of vocalic colouring in men's voices can be found in tenors. In respect to their vocal range (c – a^1) it may easily happen that the fundamental frequency is higher than the characteristic tone of the vowel *ú*. The same may be said for mezzosoprano with the vowel *ó* (g – e^2) and soprano up to *á* (b – g^2).

In research of the sung vowels it is always necessary to recognize two levels, the level of the voice and sound. Voice like all sounds has features of pitch, intensity and colour. Similarly each vowel pronounced loud has a specific pitch, intensity and colour of the voice, and in addition its own specific colour, i.e. an acoustic structure which is characteristic for the vowel.

Experiments were carried on test subject RV (tenor, professional singer) to discover how different intensities affect the colour of the vowel. The results indicate that vowel colour in the individual vowels remains constant much longer with changes in pitch if they are realized pianissimo, than at forte or fortissimo. This same followed from experiments with test subject MN (soprano).

The relatively small number of sound changes in the material examined is explained by the fact that the test subjects were realizing the vowels in syllables or monosyllabic words, so that they were able to devote much greater concentration to the articulation than to singing the texts. It can be seen that there are various individual prerequisites for the compensation of two opposing tendencies which are present in singing, i.e. maintenance of the prescribed basic tone when within the formant domain of another vowel, and preservation of the vocalic colour of the vowel to be realised. For the professional singer and for the study of bel canto the solution of this problem has great importance.

3. MUSCULAR TONUS OF THE ARTICULATORY ORGANS IN PHONATION

Already in the initial analyses of static X-ray films of the articulatory shape of the speech-organs during phonation made in 1956 we observed changes in the shape of the soft parts of the speech-organs from which we can judge that during articulation there are varying degrees of muscular tension of the soft palate, the tongue and the rear wall of the throat.[13] Analyses of films taken by serial roentgenography represent even more objective material for the evaluation of muscular tension (tonus) in the organs of articulation during phonation. The completest foundation for the evaluation of the dynamic relating in the supraglottal cavities throughout the phonatory process is afforded by cineradiographic shots of the organs of articulation during phonation.

12 *Akustika* 1903, p. 161.

13 According to comparative analysis of the cineradiographic films we designate muscular tonus from the scale: very weak, mild, strong and very strong. The use of electromyography, which affords exact results, has of course a strong influence on natural articulation. See for example R. Husson, "Vznik hlasu z hlediska elektroakustického", *SO* 22 (1961) 213-221.

If we compare overall cineradiographic shots of the soft parts of the articulatory organs without phonation, with shots of their movements during phonation, we find a marked difference and changes in their muscular tension. These differences between the muscular tenseness and muscular relaxation take place very rapidly and produce the impression of mutual parting of the soft palate and the tongue (during phonation) and coming together (in the phase without phonation). When there is a muscular relaxation (e.g. before phonation) the tongue and the soft palate come together; with an increase of muscular tension their shape changes and as a rule they move apart from each other.

Cineradiographic films show that by the smallest fraction of a second before the voice is heard the soft palate is lifted at great speed up to the level of the hard palate. As the voice is heard the soft palate and the uvula reach the culminatory phase in the articulation of the given vowel, which with the different test subjects has a different form within the framework of the characteristic position for the given vowel. In some persons the muscular tension causes the soft palate and the uvula to be raised, thickened and pressed to the rear wall of the pharynx; in other persons the muscular tension is seen in the movement of the uvula towards the oral cavity. On the other hand in some persons, even with strong muscular tension in the soft palate, the uvula was lowered and directed towards the throat cavity.

As phonation of the vowel is completed the soft palate again abandons its articulatory form a fraction of a second earlier than the tongue. The movement of the soft palate and the uvula confirms the cooperation of the speech organs during articulation. Cineradiographic films show that it is inappropriate to speak of the 'position' or the 'fixed formation' of the speech-organs during the phonation of a given vowel because not even with long vowels is the respective disposition of the soft parts entirely constant throughout the period of phonation.

The tonus of the soft palate and the tongue is in a varying intensity relation, characteristic for each specific vowel. During the vowel *í* the tonus of the soft palate is higher than that of the tongue though with *ú* the tonus of the tongue is greater than that of the soft palate; in the realisation of the vowel *á* the tonus of the tongue and of the soft palate are both medium. In the sequence of articulation working from the front vowels to the back vowels, i.e. in the direction *í*, *é*, *ó*, *ú*, there is gradual increase in muscular tension of the tongue, and that of the soft palate decreases. The muscular tension of the rear wall of the throat is manifested in the marked contraction and deviation of Passavant's cushion forward towards the tense and thickened soft palate.[14] In this way are produced the various degrees of velopharyngeal closure or passage.[15]

14 Marked individual differences are observed in the functioning of Passavante's cushion. "According to the different positions of the soft palate are formed:

(a) an absolutely free entrance to the nose cavity: with easy breathing... (b) an only partially freed entrance; the soft palate is not lowered so far as with absolutely easy breathing, but remains somewhat raised and prepared for the articulation of the following sound; these are either the vowels

Let us look more closely at how the velopharyngeal closure or passage appears with a change in intensity.

With PIANISSIMO there was a velopharyngeal closure when *í* was realised by the second and third persons. A clear passage was observed in the first person. When *é* was articulated there was a clear passage to the nasal cavity in the first subject, in the second the soft palate touches the rear wall of the throat, and in the third there was a velopharyngeal closure. In the articulation of the vowel *á* the first subject showed quite a wide velopharyngeal passage, in the second subject no contact was made between the soft palate and the rear wall of the throat, and in the third person there was a weak velopharyngeal closure. The articulation of *ó* was realised by the first person with quite a wide passage to the nasal cavity, by the second with a narrow gap, and by the third with a velopharyngeal closure. The first subject showed again a quite wide velopharyngeal passage in the realisation of *ú;* in the second person there was no contact of the soft palate with the rear wall of the throat, and the third produced a velopharyngeal closure.

During the realisation of the vowels at MEZZOFORTE (medium intensity) the relationships in the velopharyngeal area were as follows: with the articulation of *í* the first person showed a velopharyngeal gap, the second a velopharyngeal closure. With the vowel *é* it was possible to observe in the first person a velopharyngeal gap to the nasal cavity; the second person produced a velopharyngeal closure, and in the third person the muscular tension was also less than at pianissimo. With the vowel *á* there was a velopharyngeal gap in the first person, the second made the closure, and in the third there was less muscular tension than at pianissimo. When *ó* was realised a wide velopharyngeal gap was visible in the first person, the second showed a velopharyngeal closure, and in the third there was once more less muscular tension than at pianissimo.

When pronouncing *ú* the first person made a velopharyngeal gap, the second a velopharyngeal closure, and in the third person the muscular tension was again less than at pianissimo.

At FORTISSIMO the velopharyngeal closure was produced in all three test subjects for the vowel *í*. With *é* there was a passage to the nasal cavity in the first subject, in the second the velopharyngeal closure was effected, and in the third there was but slight contact. The vowel *á* produced a passage to the nasal cavity in the first subject,

---

called nasal vowels or nasals (in French, Portuguese, and Polish) or the consonants m, n, ň (nasal consonants)... (c) a further manner of articulation is a partial vibration of the edges of the soft palate during the so-called back, velar *r*; however there also exists an *r* made by the vibration of the uvula in the narrow opening between the tongue and the soft palate (uvular *r*). (d) The final possibility is a velopharyngeal closure which is formed with all non-nasal sounds. This closure has not always the same strength. Of the vowels *i* and *u* have the strongest closure, *a* the weakest, and with *e* and *o* it is of medium strength..." (B. Hála – M. Sovák, *Hlas – řeč – sluch*, Praha, 1962[4], p. 99).

[15] H. H. Wängler in "Über die Funktion des weichen Gaumens beim Sprechen", (*WZ* 11 [1962] 1747-1751) comes to conclusions, for German vowels similar to our results for Czech vowels. These are to be found in the thesis of J. Ondráčková, "Artikulace českých zpívaných samohlásek", 1960 (thesis.)

in the second a velopharyngeal closure, and in the third there was weak contact. With the vowel *ó* the first person showed a passage to the nasal cavity, the second a velopharyngeal closure and in the third case it was not possible to demonstrate safely the passage to the nasal cavity. With *ú* there was a velopharyngeal closure in the second subject. The first and third articulated *ú* as strongly coloured towards *ó*.

The material investigated indicates that precisely various degrees of muscular tension and their respective combinations among the individual articulatory organs are relevant for the formation of the conditions necessary for the specific articulatory form of a particular vowel. Muscular tension of the soft palate grows with a deviation from the middle intensities and frequencies both up and down, in speech and in singing.

If the soft palate has the most active share in making a tight velopharyngeal closure, one might assume that the tightness of the closure is directly proportional to the muscular tension of the soft palate, or in reverse that an increase in the muscular tension of the soft palate has the effect of intensifying the velopharyngeal closure. The films show however that even in the presence of quite strong tonus in the soft palate, the formation of the velopharyngeal closure is not automatic.

For the ability to form a velopharyngeal closure the muscular tension of the soft palate and the rear wall of the throat is more important than the length of the soft palate.[16]

Cineradiographic films showing the dynamics of the articulatory process demonstrate quite clearly that in many cases there arises a fluctuation in the degree of muscular tension in the rear wall of the throat and the soft palate by which the width of the passage to the nasal cavity or the firmness of the velopharyngeal closure during the phonation of the same vowel may vary without these fine articulatory changes being detectable to the ear i.e. one cannot evaluate the vowel as nasalised as a result of a direct connection to the nasal cavity. From this it follows that it is inappropriate to state the presence or absence of the velopharyngeal closure as one of the basic properties by which to evaluate Czech long vowels. The detected changes in the firmness of the velopharyngeal closure, which may change even during the same vowel, are either too rapid to be manifested auditively, or this fine articulatory movement comes within the tolerance range of the identifiability of the vowel. This is supported by the fact that in the material investigated there were various degrees of velopharyngeal closures and passages.[17] Not even during the singing of the scale up and down could the neutral vowel which was realised be differently evaluated in the moment of close approach of the soft palate to the rear wall of the throat as against its realisation when it moved away from the rear wall of the throat. From this it

[16] Knowledge of the method of the physiological formation of the velopharyngeal closure is of great importance for overcoming imperfect functional dynamics of the soft palate. Cf. e.g. M. H. L. Hecker, "Studies of Nasal Consonants with an Articulatory Speech Synthesizer", *JASA* 34 (1962) 179-188.

[17] Confr e.g. H. Mol's investigations of nasality.

follows that it is not a necessary prerequisite for a Czech vowel to be assessed from the acoustic point of view as non-nasal that there be an unconditional realisation of the velopharyngeal closure during its articulation. Czech long vowels can be evaluated according to the material analysed as *vowels inclining to a varying degree of velopharyngeal closure or passage*. This instability in the formation of the passage or closure corresponds to the fact that in Czech there is no opposition of nasal and non-nasal vowels. Nasality can not be understood as a phenomenon having quantitatively the same marks in different languages.

REFERENCES

Abramson, A. S. and F. S. Cooper.
1963 "Slow-motion X-ray Pictures with Stretched Speech as a Research Tool", *JASA* 35, 1888-89.
Artemov, V. A.
1956 *Eksperimentalnaja fonetika* (Moskva).
Aulich, J.
1961 "Fotoelektrické odpory spékané s přívodními elektrodami", *SO* 22, 397-401.
Berg, J. van den.
1955a "Calculations on a Model of the Vocal Tract for Vowel /i/ /meat/ and of the Larynx", *JASA* 27, 332-38.
1955b "Transmission of the Vocal Cavities", JASA 27, 161-68.
Björk, L.
1961 "Velopharyngeal Function in Connected Speech", *ARS Supplementum* 202.
Bjuggren, G. and G. Fant.
1964 "The Nasal Cavity Structures", *STL-QPSR* 4:5.
Boy, M., H. Lühmann, and J. Schweinitz.
1961 *Foto und Filmtechnik in der Medizin* (Halle: Saale).
Brombart, M.
1962 "Clinical Radiology of the Esophagus", *AJR* 88, 384-85.
Calnan, J. S.
1953 "Movements of the Soft Palate", *British Journal of Plastic Surgery* 5, 286-96.
Calzia-Panconcelli, G.
1919 "Phonetische Röntgenpolygramme", *Vox* 29, 170-79.
Carmody, F. J.
1941 "An X-ray Study of Pharyngeal Articulation", *UCPMPh* 21, 377-84.
Chiba, I. and M. Kajiyama
1941 *The Vowel, Its Nature and Structure* (Tokyo).
Chlumský, J.
1928 *Česká kvantita, melodie a přízvuk* (Praha).
Chlumský, J., A. Pauphilet, and B. Polland.
1938 *Radiografie francouzských samohlásek a polosamohlásek* (Praha).
Clerk, J. L. de, et al.
1965 "Cinefluorography of the Vocal Part", *5th I. C. A., Liège*, Rap. A26, 1-4.
Coleman, R. O.
1965 "The Effect of Changes in Width of Velopharyngeal Aperture on Acoustic and Perceptual Properties of Nasalized Vowels", *Linguistics* 12, 102-04.
Croatto, L.
1960 "L'intervention du doublement de la paroi postérieur du pharynx comme complément à la chirurgie réparatrice du palais et dans les insuffisances vélaires", *FPh Supplement*, 55-63.
Croatto, L. and C. Croatto-Martinolli.
1959 "Physiopathologie du voile du palais", *FPh* 11, 124-66.
Curry, R.
1938 "The Physiology of the Contralto Voice", *ANPE* 14, 73-79.

Czermak, J.
1879 *Über das Verhalten des weichen Gaumens beim Hervorbringen der reinen Vokale* (Leipzig).
Čistovič, L. et al.
1968 "Psychological Methods in Speech Perception Research", *ZPhSK* 21, 33-39.
Damsté, P. H.
1962 "Cineradiographic Observations of Velar and Glottal Movements", *Proceedings of the 4th International Congress of Phonetic Sciences, Helsinki 1961* (The Hague), 147-48.
1968 "X-ray Study of Phonation", *Proceedings of the 14th International Congress of Logopedics and Phoniatrics* (Paris), 65-68.
Delattre, P.
1954 "Les attributs acoustiques de la nasalité vocalique et consonantique", *Studia Linguistica* 2, 103-09.
Dieth, E.
1950 *Vademekum der Phonetik* (Bern).
Elbert, M., R. L. Schelton, and W. B. Arndt.
1967 "A Task for Evaluation of Articulation Change: 1. Development of Methodology", *JSHR* 10, 281-88.
Essen, O. von.
1953 *Allgemeine und angewandte Phonetik* (Berlin).
Fant, G.
1960 *Acoustic Theory of Speech Production* (The Hague).
1965 "Formants and Cavities", *Proceedings of the 5th International Congress of Phonetic Sciences, Münster 1964* (Basel-New York), 120-41.
Fischer-Jørgensen, E. and A. T. Hansen.
1959 "An Electrical Manometer and its Use in Phonetic Research", *Ph* 4, 43-53.
Flanagan, J. L.
1965 *Speech Analysis, Synthesis and Perception* (Berlin).
Fritzell, B.
1969 *The Velopharyngeal Muscles in Speech* (Göteborg).
Fröschels, E.
1920 *Singen und Sprechen, ihre Anatomie, Physiologie und Hygiene* (Leipzig-Wien).
Fujimura, O.
1962 "Analysis of Nasal Consonants", *JASA* 34, 1865-75.
Gottheiner, V. and E. Zwirner.
1933 "Die Verwendung des Röntgentonfilms für die Sprachforschung", *FGR* 17, 455-62.
Gutzmann, H.
1930 "Röntgenaufnahmen von Zunge und Gaumensegel bei Vokalen und Dauerkonsonanten", *FGR* 41, 392-404.
Hála, B.
1941 *Akustická podstata somohlásek* (Praha).
1960 *Fonetické obrazy hlásek* (Praha).
1962 *Uvedení do fonetiky češtiny na obecně fonetickém základě* (Praha).
Hála, B. and M. Sovák.
1962 *Hlas-řeč-sluch* (Praha).
Hecker, M. H. L.
1962 "Studies of Nasal Consonants with an Articulatory Speech Synthesizer", *JASA* 34, 179-88.
Hegedüs, L.
1937 "Roentgenaufnahmen von ungarischen Vokalen", *ANPE* 13, 72-77.
Heinz, J. M.
1967 "Perturbation Functions for the Determination of Vocal-tract Eigenvalues", *STL-QPSR* 1, 1-14.
Heinz, J. M. and K. N. Stevens.
1965 "On the Relations between Lateral Cineradiograph Area Functions and Acoustic Spectra of Speech", *5th I. C. A. Liège*, Rap. A44, 1-5.

Hermann, L.
1911 "Neue Beiträge zur Lehre von den Vokalen und ihrer Entstehung", *Pflüger's Archiv für die gesammte Physiologie* 141.
Holbrook, R. T. and F. J. Carmody.
1937 "X-ray Studies of Speech Articulations", *UCPMPh* 20.
Honegger, A.
1952 *Ich bin Komponist* (Zürich).
House, A. S. and K. N. Stevens.
1956 "Analog Studies of the Nasalisation of Vowels", *JSHD* 21, 218-32.
Husson, R.
1959 "Der gegenwärtige Stand der physiologischen Phonetik", *Ph* 4, 1-32.
1960 *La voix chantée* (Paris).
1961 "Vznik hlasu z hlediska elektroakustického", *SO* 22, 213-21.
1962 *La physiologie de la phonation* (Paris).
Jacobson, H. and J. H. Shapiro.
1959 "Simultaneous Biplane Large Seriography in Cerebral Angiography", *AJR* 82, 773-78.
Jakobson, R. and M. Halle
1956 *Fundamentals of Language* (The Hague).
Jakobson, R., G. Fant, and M. Halle.
1955 *Preliminaries to Speech Analysis* (Cambridge, Mass.).
Janker, R.
1945 *Röntgenaufnahmetechnik* (Leipzig).
Janota, P.
1949 *K otázce měření dynamiky řeči* (thesis).
1967 *Personal Characteristics of Speech* (Praha).
Janota, P. and L. Švestková
1959 "K metodice výzkumu retní činnosti", *AUC – Philologica*, 37-44.
Jones, D.
1950 *The Phoneme; Its Nature and Use* (Cambridge).
Judin, S. P.
1956 *Pevec i golos.*
Kaňka, F.
1927 *Podmínky umělých samohláskových zvuků* (Praha).
Kiml, J.
1962 "Trouble de la voix dans le sillon des cordes vocales", *FPh* 14, 272-79.
Kirkpatrick, J. A. and R. W. Olmsted.
1959 "Cinefluorographic Study of Pharyngeal Function Related to Speech", *R* 73, 557-59.
Kloster-Jensen, M.
1970 "Physiologie et enseignement de la prononciation", *International Review of Applied Linguistics in Language Teaching* 8, 221-25.
Koneczna, H. and W. Zawadowski.
1956 *Obrazy rentgenograficzne głosek rosyjskich* (Warszawa).
Krech, H.
1957 "Hochlautung und Kunstgesang", *WZ* 6:5, 883-89.
1960 "Über ein einfaches Verfahren zur Aufzeichnung des oralen und nasalen Schalldruckanteils gesprochener Sprache", *FPh Supplement* 1, 100-08.
Ladefoged, P.
1967 *Three Areas of Experimental Phonetics* (London).
Lane, H.
1971 "Production et perception de la parole. Rapports et différences", *Ph* 23, 94-125.
Leden, H. van, P. Moore, and R. Timcke.
1960 "Laryngeal Vibrations: Measurements of the Glottic Wave", *AO* 71, 16-35.
Lehiste, I.
1970 *Suprasegmentals* (Cambridge, Mass. and London).

Liberman, A. M., F. S. Cooper, K. S. Harris, and P. F. MacNeilage.
1962 "A Motor Theory of Speech Perception", Speech Communication Seminar 2, Stockholm, 29 August-1 September.
Lieberman, P.
1967 *Intonation, Perception, and Language* (Cambridge, Mass.).
Liiv, G. and A. Eek.
1968 "Some Notes on Experimental Research Problems in Speech Production Dynamics (with Special Reference to Complex Techniques of Cinefluorography Synchronized with Sound Spectrography)", *Izvestija akademii nauk estonskej SSR* 17, biologia, 78-102.
Lindblom, B.
1965 "Dynamic Aspects of Vowel Articulation", *Proceedings of the 5th International Congress of Phonetic Sciences, Münster 1964* (The Hague), 387-88.
Lindblom, B. and P. O. Bivner.
1966 "A Method for Continuous Recording of Articulatory Movement", *STL-QPSR* 1, 14-16.
Lindner, G.
1969a *Einführung in die experimentelle Phonetik* (Berlin).
1969b "Theoretische Analyse des Sprechbewegungsablaufs", *ZPhSK* 22, 450-73.
Lindqvist, J. and S. E. Öhman.
1966 "Instrumentation for Subglottal and Supraglottal Air Pressure Measurements", *STL-QPSR* 1, 9-10.
Lindqvist, J. and S. Pauli.
1968 "The Role of Relative Spectrum Levels in Vowel Perception", *STL-QPSR* 2:3, 12-15.
Lubker, J. F. and J. F. Curtis.
1966 "Electromyographic-cinefluorographic Investigation of Velar Function During Speech Production", *JASA* 40, 1272.
Lubker, J. F. and H. L. Morris.
1968 "Predicting Cinefluorographic Measures of Velopharyngeal Opening from Lateral Still X-ray Films", *JSHR* 11, 747-53.
Luchsinger, R.
1953 "Physiologie der Stimme", *FPh* 5, 58-127.
Macmillan, A. S. and G. Kelemen.
1952 "Radiography of the Supraglottic Speech Organs", *AO* 55, 671-88.
Malécot, A.
1960 "Vowel Nasality as a Distinctive Feature in American English", *Language* 36, 222-29.
Malmberg, B.
1964 *New Trends in Linguistics* (Stockholm).
Malmberg, B., ed.
1968 *Manual of Phonetics* (Amsterdam).
Martóny, J.
1964 "The Role of Formant Amplitudes in Synthesis of Nasal Consonants", *STL-QPSR* 3, 28-31.
Massengill, R., Jr.
1967 "A Study of Velopharyngeal Function as Related to Perceived Nasality of Vowels, Utilizing a Cinefluorographic Television Monitor", *FPh* 19, 45-52.
Mattson, O.
1952 "Aspects of the Interpretation of Contrast and Detail in Radiographs", *ARS* 38, 477-88.
McDonnel, G. M., H. L. Berman, and E. A. Lodmell.
1958 "Supervoltage Roentgenography", *AJR* 79, 306-20.
McGinnis, C. S., M. Elnick, and M. Kraichman.
1951 "A Study of the Vowel Formants of Well-known Male Operatic Singers", *JASA* 23, 440-46.
Mechanizmy Rečeobrazovanija i vosprijatija složnych zvukov (Problemy fiziologičeskoj akustiki V) (Moskva, Leningrad, 1966).
Meyer, E. A.
1907 "Röntgenologische Lautbilder", *MM* 17, 224-43.
Miller, E. R.
1959 "Cinefluorography in Practice", *R* 73, 560-64.

Minifie, F. D., T. J. Hixon, Ch. A. Kelsey, and R. J. Woodhouse.
1970 "Lateral Pharyngeal Wall Movement During Speech Production", *JSHR* 13, 584-94.
Mitrinowicz-Modrzejewska, A. and St. Kruszewski.
1961 "Röntgenkinematographie und die Pathologie der Stimme", *FPh* 13, 164-73.
Mol, H.
1962 "Aural Stimuli and Their Interpretation", *Proceedings of the 4th International Congress of Phonetic Sciences, Helsinki 1961* (The Hague), 320-29.
Moll, K. L.
1960 "Cinefluorographic Techniques in Speech Research", *JSHR* 3, 227-41.
Moll, K. L. and R. G. Daniloff.
1971 "Investigation of the Timing of Velar Movements During Speech", *JASA* 50, 678-84.
Neilage, P. F., J. L. de Clerk, and S. I. Silverman.
1966 "Some Relations Between Articulator Movement and Motor Control in Consonant-Vowel-Consonant Monosyllables", *JASA* 40, 1272.
Ohnesorg, K. and O. Švarný
1955 "Études expérimentales des articulations chinoises", *Rozpravy ČSAV* 65.
Ondráčková, J.
1959a "První rentgenokinematografický záznam z oblasti fonetiky češtiny", *Bulletin ČSAV* 5, 8.
1959b *The Movement of the Tongue and the Soft Palate During Singing of Vowels.* X-ray sound film.
1959c "Zpráva o první celostátní konferenci o výchově pěveckých kádrů", *NŘ* 39, 107-08.
1960a *Activity of the Soft Palate During Phonation – Direct Shots.* Color sound film.
1960b *Artikulace českých zpívaných samohlásek*, dis.
1960c "První rentgenokinematografický záznam artikulace českých zpívaných vokálů", *Věstník ČSAV* 69, 125-26.
1961a *Articulatory Movements of the Tongue and the Soft Palate – Direct Shots.* Color sound film.
1961b "The Movement of the Tongue and the Soft Palate in the Singing of Vowels", *FPh* 13, 99-106.
1962 "Objektivní analýzy rentgenogramů mluvidel", *Věstník ČSAV* 71, 558-59.
1964a "The Muscular Tension in the Superglottal Speech-Organs", *ZPhSK* 17, 257-63.
1964b "Objective Analytical Method of Roentgenograms of the Organs of Speech", *International Association of Logopedics and Phoniatrics, Proceedings of the 12th International Speech and Voice Therapy Conference, Padua, 1962*, 563-65.
1964c *Rentgenologický výzkum articulace českých vokálů* (Praha).
1964d "Zur Untersuchung der physiologischen Tätigkeit der Sprechorganen in den suppraglottischen Höhlen", *FPh* 16, 161-71.
1965a "Některé metody komplexního výzkumu fyziologie činosti mluvidel", *SaS* 26, 45-50.
1965b "On the Roentgenography of Speech Organs", *Proceedings of the 5th International Congress of Phonetic Sciences, Münster 1964* (Basel-New York), 446-49.
1965c "Zur direkten Beobachtung der Tätigkeit des weichen Gaumens", *De therapia vocis et loquellae, Societas Internationalis Logopediae et Phoniatriae, XIII. Congressus Vindobonae Anno MCMLXV*, Acta II, 117-19.
1966 "K otázce nazálního zabarvení českých samohlásek", *SaS* 27, 127-32.
1968 "P. Simon, *Les consonnes françaises*", review in *Ph* 18, 188-91.
1969 "Some Remarks on the Analysis of Sung Vowels (X-ray Study on Czech Material)", *Study of Sounds* 14, 407-18. (Phonetic Society of Japan, Tokyo).
1970 "The Velopharyngeal Passage in View of Nasality (X-ray Study)", *Procédés des Séances du 14e Congrès of Logopedics and Phoniatrics, Paris 1968* (Paris), 497-503.
Ondráčková, J., J. Lindqvist, and G. Fant.
1970 "Electrical Glottography", *Proceedings of the 6th International Congress of Phonetic Sciences, Prague 1967* (Prague), 709-11.
Ondráčková, J. and R. Poch.
1957 "Zur Methodik der Untersuchung der Vokalartikulation beim Gesang", *ZPhS* 10, 258-68.
1962a "Nativní rentgenokinematografie mluvidel", *ČR* 16, 92-99.
1962b "New Roentgenographic Methods in the Research of the Activity of the Articulatory Organs", *IJR* 16, 137-50.

Onishi, M.
1970 "Perception of Quality Versus Quantity", *Proceedings of the 6th International Congress of Phonetic Sciences, Prague 1967* (Prague), 713-715.
Öhman, S. E.
1965 "X-ray Studies of Articulatory Dynamics", *Proceedings of the 5th International Congress of Phonetic Sciences, Münster 1964* (Basel-New York), 16-23.
1966 "Coarticulation in VCV Utterances: Spectrographic Measurements", *JASA* 39, 151-68.
Öhman, S. E. and K. N. Stevens.
1963 "Cineradiographic Studies of Speech: Procedures and Objectives", *JASA* 35, 1889.
Palatolalie (Praha, 1956).
Perelló, J.
1960 "Contribution casuistique à la pathologie du voile du palais", *FPh* 12, 113-17.
Parmenter, C. E., S. N. Treviño, and C. A. Bevans.
1931 "A Technique for Radiographing the Organs of Speech During Articulation", *ZEPh* 1, 63-84.
Perkell, J. S.
1965 "Cinematographic Studies of Speech: Implications of a Detailed Analysis of Certain Articulatory Movements", *5th I. C. A.*, Liège.
Peterson, G. E. and H. L. Barney.
1952 "Control Methods Used in a Study of the Vowels", *JASA* 24, 175-84.
Pfau, W.
1962 "Chronaxie und Stimmgattung", *FPh* 14, 1-14.
Pike, K. L.
1967 "Tongue-root Position in Practical Phonetics", *Ph* 17, 129-40.
Pimonow, L., P. Pouteaux, and R. Husson.
1960 "Modifications des spectres acoustiques et absorbtion exercées par le pavillion pharyngobucconasal pendant la phonation", *Comptes rendus des séances de l'Académie des Sciences* 251, 280-82.
Poch, R. and J. Ondráčková.
1966 "Rentgenokinematografie", *Film ve vysokoškolské výuce* (Praha), 125-34.
Polland, B. and B. Hála.
1926 *Artikulace českých zvuků v roentgenových obrazech (skiagramech)* (Praha).
Přecechtěl, A., R. Hladký, F. Kotyza, and K. Sedláček.
1959 *Základy otolaryngologie* (Praha).
Reformatskij, A. A.
1955 *Reč i muzyka v penii* (Moskva).
Romportl, M.
1953 "Fonetická studie o ruském ы" *Slavia* 22, 529-56.
1957 "Neuer Beitrag zur slavischen Phonetik", *ZPhS* 10, 289-93.
Romportl, M. and P. Janota.
1959 "Ein Beitrag zur phonetischen Methodik (Die Gehöranalyse als Bestandtteil der experimentelphonetischen Forschung)", *AUC – Philologica* 1, 17-28.
Rubin, H. J., M. Le Cover, and W. Vennard.
1967 "Vocal Intensity, Subglottic Pressure and Air Flow Relationships in Singers", *FPh* 19, 393-413.
Russel, G. O.
1934 "First Preliminary X-ray Consonant Study", *JASA* 5, 247-51.
Russel, G. O. and J. Palomo.
1934 "Synchronized X-ray and Oscillographic Records", *JASA* 5, 223.
Scheier, M.
1909 "Die Bedeutung des Röntgensverfahrens für die Physiologie der Sprache und der Stimme", *ALR* 22, 175-208.
Sedláček, K.
1956 *Základy audiologie* (Praha).
1962 "Akustická analýza zpěvního hlasu", ČLČ 101, 291-96.

Sedláček, K. and A. Synchra.
1962 *Hudba a slovo z experimentálního hlediska* (Praha).
Simon, P.
1967 *Les consonnes françaises (mouvements et positions articulatoires à la lumière de la radiocinématographie)* (Paris).
Shelton, R. L., W. B. Arndt, A. W. Knox, M. Elbert, L. Chisum, and K. A. Joungstrom.
1969 "The Relationship between Nasal Sound Pressure Level and Palatopharyngeal Closure", *JSHR* 12, 193-98.
Skaličková, A.
1955 "The Korean Vowels", *Archiv orientální*, 23 (Praha).
Smith, S.
1957 "Chest Register Versus Head Register in the Membrane Cushion Model of the Vocal Cords", *FPh* 9, 32-36.
Sonesson, B.
1968 "The Functional Anatomy of the Speech Organs", in B. Malmberg, ed., *Manual of Phonetics*, 45-75.
Sovijärvi, A.
1938 *Die gehaltenen, geflüsterten un gesungenen Vokale und Nasale der finnischen Sprache* (Helsinki).
1959 "Über die Veränderlichkeit der Zungenstellung und der entsprechenden akustischen Schwankungsgebiete der Vokale auf Grund eines Röntgentonfilms gesprochener finnischer Sätze", *Ph* 4, *Supplement*, 74-84.
1970 "On Transition in the Light of X-ray Films", *Proceedings of the 6th International Congress of Phonetic Sciences, Prague 1967* (Prague), 851-55.
Stevens, K. N.
1968 "On the Relations Between Speech Movements and Speech Perception", Seminar on Speech Production and Perception, Leningrad 1966, *ZPhSK* 21, 102-06.
Stevens, K. N. and A. S. House.
1963 "Perturbation of Vowel Articulation by Consonantal Context: An Acoustical Study", *JSHR* 6, 111-28.
Strouhal, Č.
1903 *Akustika* (Praha).
Subtelny, Joanne D. and J. Daniel Subtelny.
1962 "Roentgenographic Techniques and Phonetic Research", *Proceedings of the 4th International Congress of Phonetic Sciences, Helsinki 1961* (The Hague), 129-46.
Sundberg, J.
1968 "Formant Frequencies of Bass Singers", *STL-QPSR* 1, 1-6.
Tarneaud, J.
1946 *Le Chant, sa construction, sa destruction* (Paris).
Tarnóczy, T.
1943 "Resonanzdaten der Vokalresonatoren", *AZ* 8, 22-31.
Trojan, F.
1959 "Die Ausdruckstheorie der Sprechstimme", *Ph* 4, 121-50.
1960 "Zur entwicklungsgeschichtlichen Beziehung des Vokalismus zu den Registern", *APPhL* 1, 41-47.
Truby, H. M.
1959 "Acoustico-Cineradiographic Analysis: Considerations with Especial Reference to Certain Consonantal Complexes", *AR Supplement* 182, 1-227.
1962 "Synchronized Cineradiography and Visual-Acoustic Analysis", *Proceedings of the 4th International Congress of Phonetic Sciences, Helsinki 1961* (The Hague), 265-79.
Tuddenham, J. W.
1957 "The Visual Physiology of Roentgen Diagnosis", *AJR* 78, 116-23.
Ungeheuer, G.
1962 *Elemente einer akustischen Theorie der Vokal-artikulation* (Berlin).
Vallancien, B.
1960 "Cinématique de la glotte en voix chantée", *APPhL Supplement FPh* 1, 13-18.

1970 "Étude radiologique de la phonation", *Proceedings of the 14th International Congress of Logopedics and Phoniatrics, Paris 1968* (Paris), 156-81.

Wängler, H. H.
1961 *Atlas deutscher Sprachlaute* (Berlin).
1962 "Über die Funktion des weichen Gaumens beim Sprechen", *WZ* 11, 1747-51.

Wierzchowska, B. and J. Wierzchowski.
1969 "Nasal Phonemes and Their Realization in Polish", *Study of Sounds* 14, 397-406 (Phonetic Society of Japan, Tokyo).

Winter, F. S. and J. S. Lehman.
1959 "Rotational Cinefluorography", *AJR* 82, 120-24.

Wode, H.
1970 *Linguistische Untersuchungen zum Parkinsonismus* (Basel-New York).

Zwirner, E. and K. Zwirner.
1966 *Grundfragen der Phonometrie* (Basel-New York).

Žinkin, N. I.
1958 *Mechanizmy reči* (Moskva).

APPENDIX

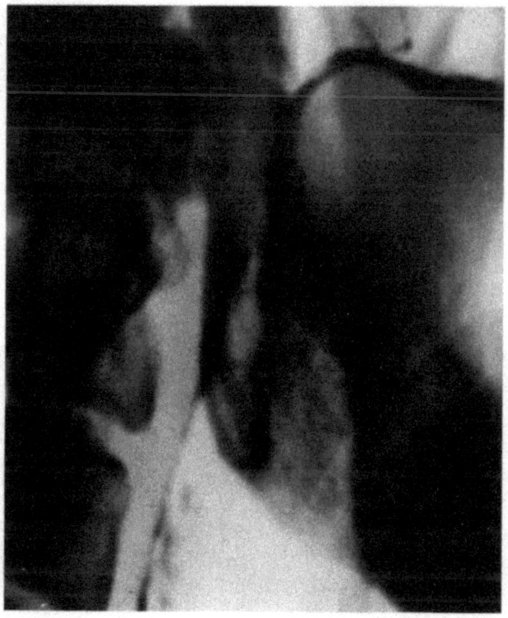

Fig. 1 – A sample of the X-ray method using barium paste as a contrast medium. The barium paste is blocking the velo-pharyngeal passage to a considerable degree.

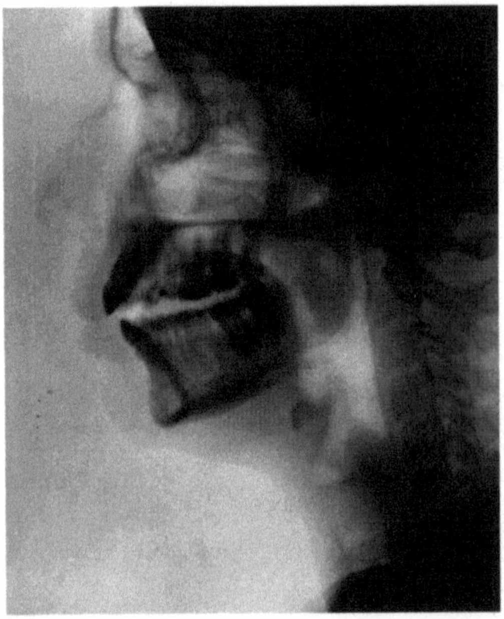

639

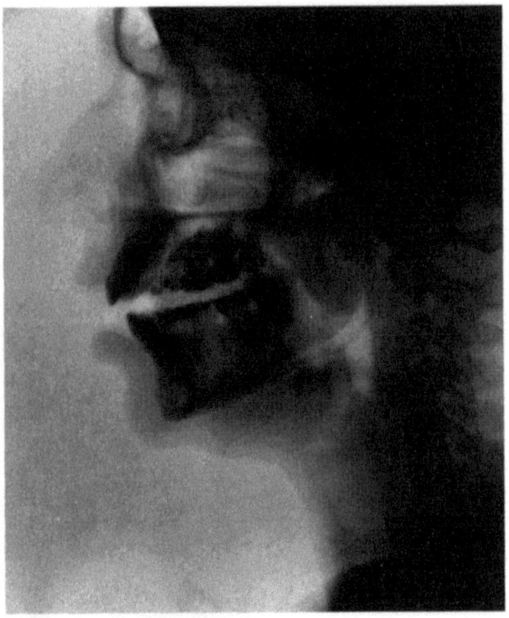

641

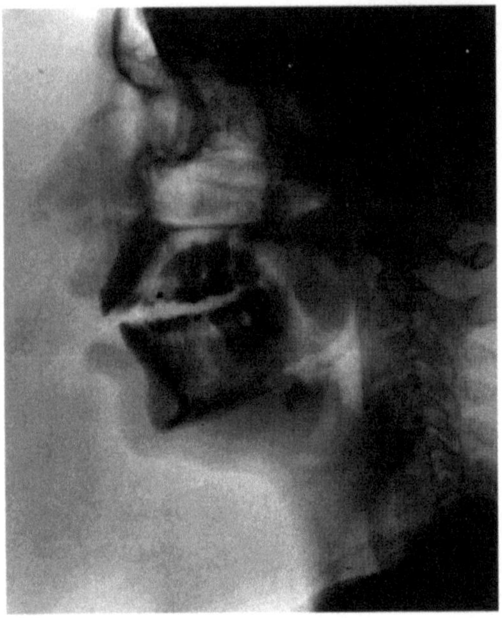

642

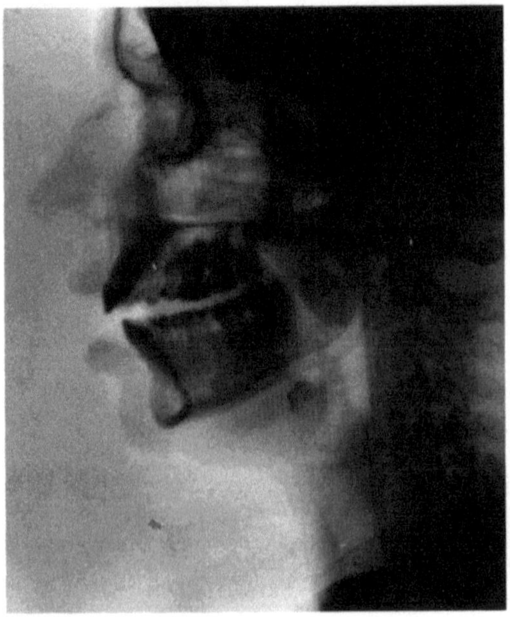

643

Fig. 2 – Pictures obtained by means of serial roentgenography without using any contrast medium. Series No. 18 /HŠ/ demonstrates the articulation of vowels sung in the syllables *bí*, *bé*, *bá*, *bó*, *bú*.
Picture 639 – the occlusion of the consonant *b*.
Pictures 641, 642, 643, 644, 645 – the articulatory phases in the singing of the vowel *í*.

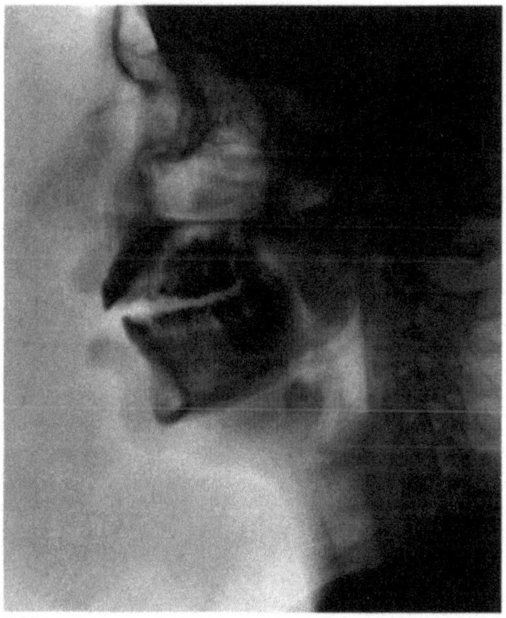
644

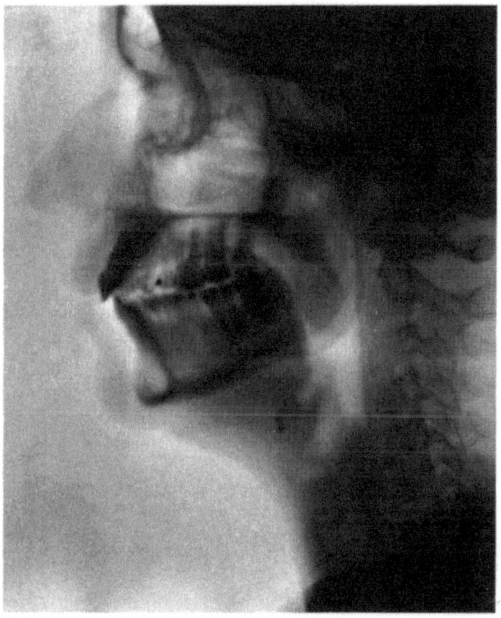
645

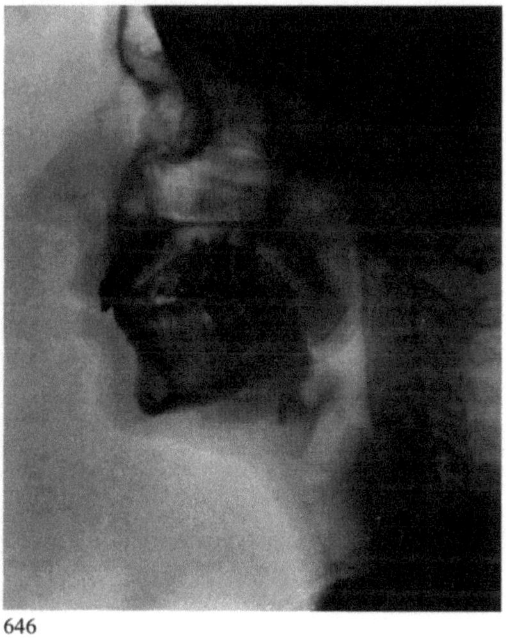
646

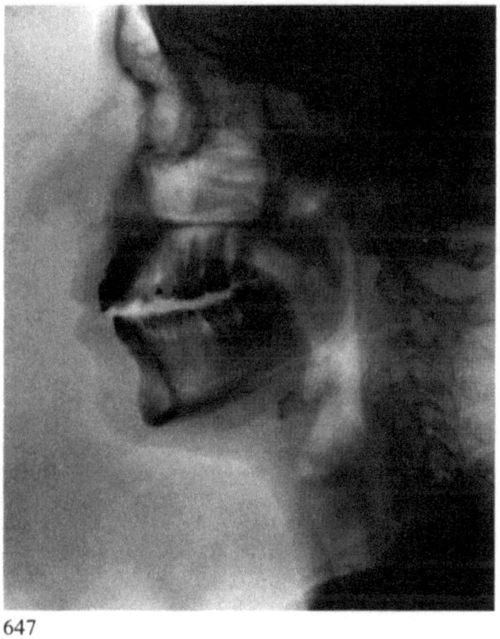
647

646 – speech organs without phonation.
647 – the occlusion of the consonant *b*.

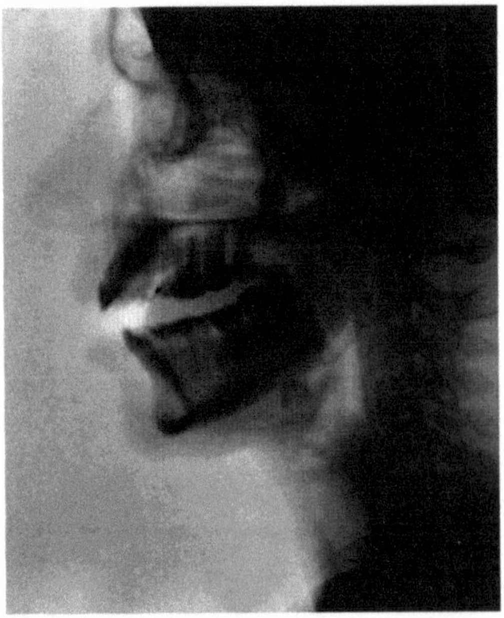

648

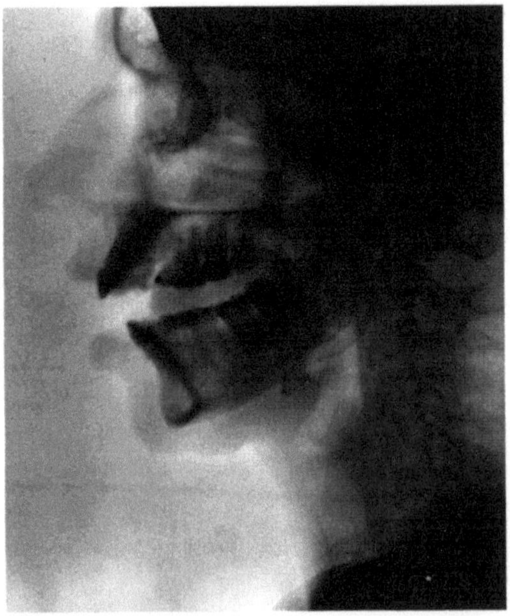

649

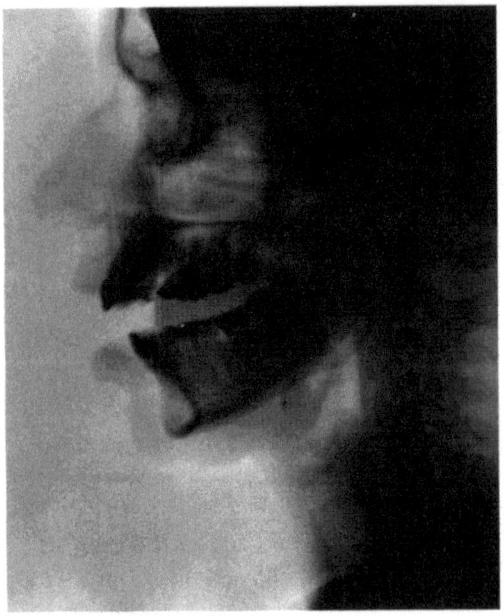

650

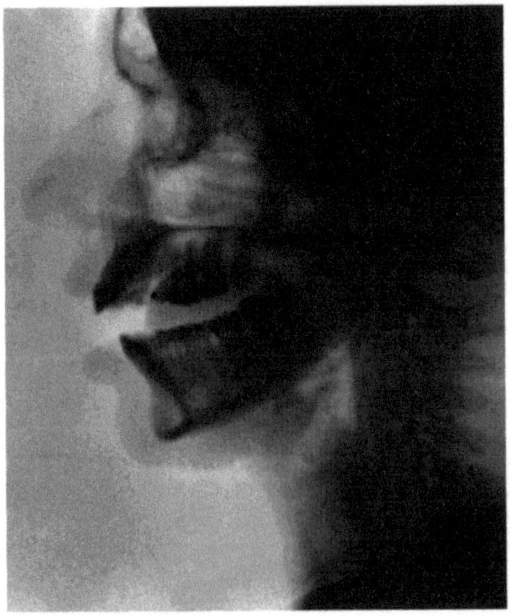

651

648, 649, 650, 651, 652, 653 – the articulatory phases in the singing of the vowel *é*.

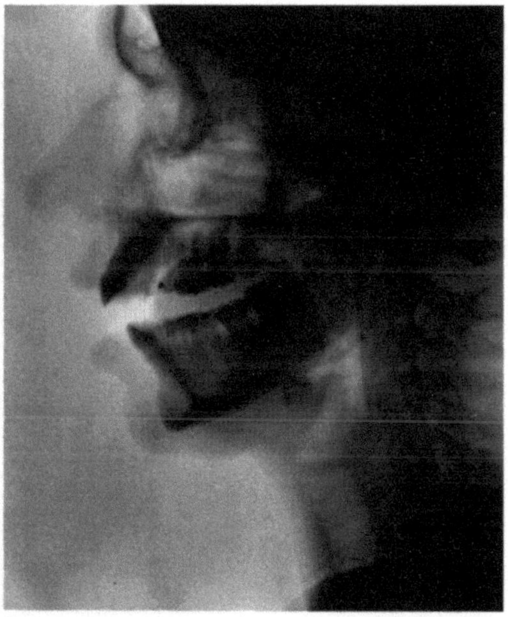
652

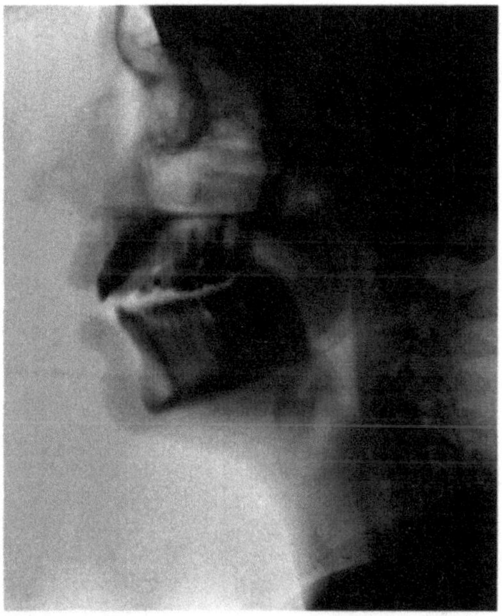
653

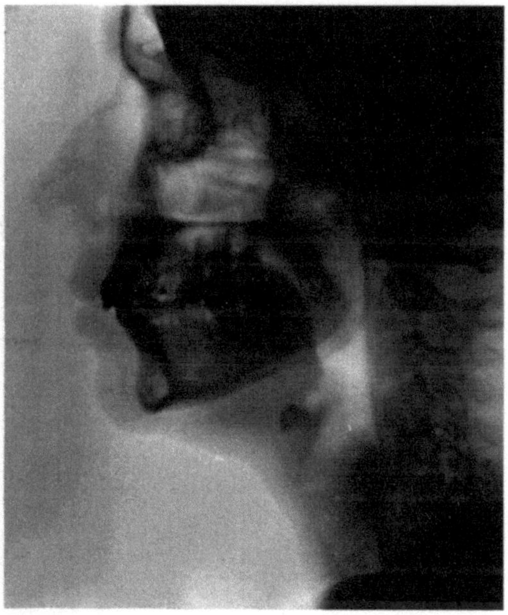
654

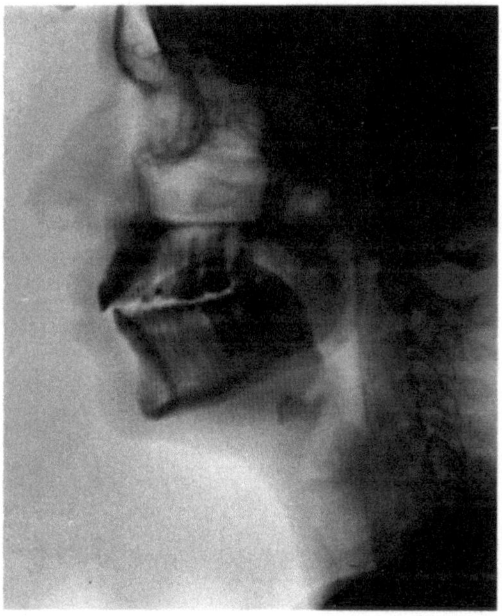
655

654 – speech organs without phonation.
655 – the occlusion of the consonant *b*.

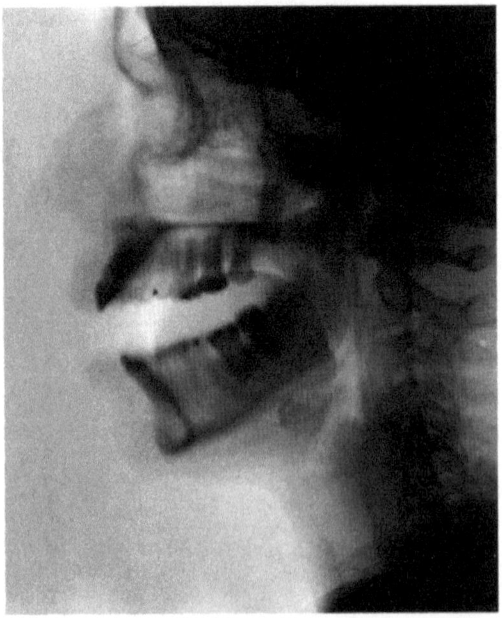

656

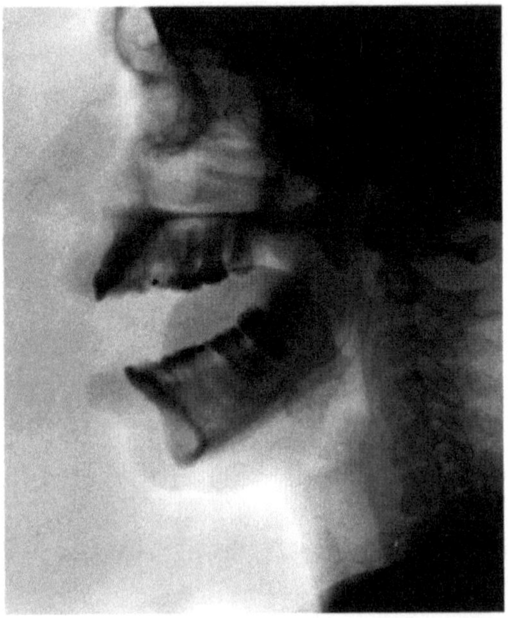

657

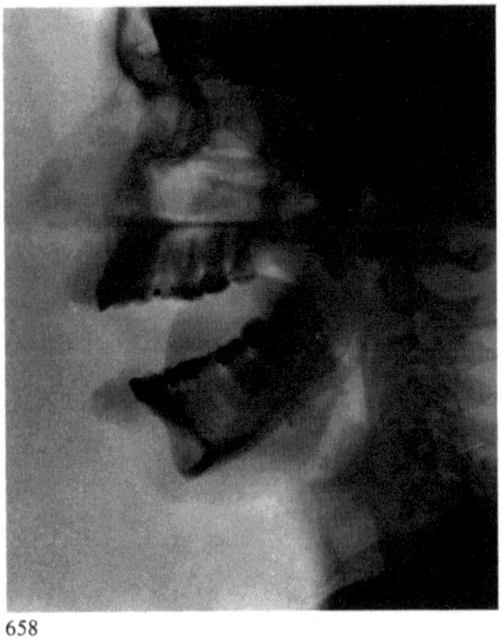

658

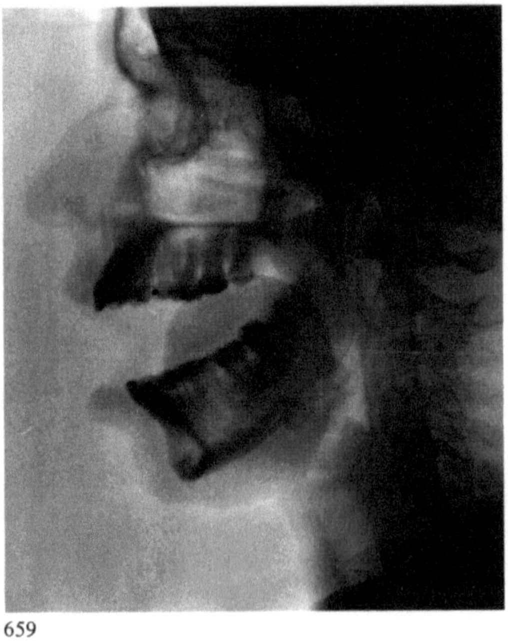

659

656, 657, 658, 659, 660 – the articulatory phases in the singing of the vowel *á*.

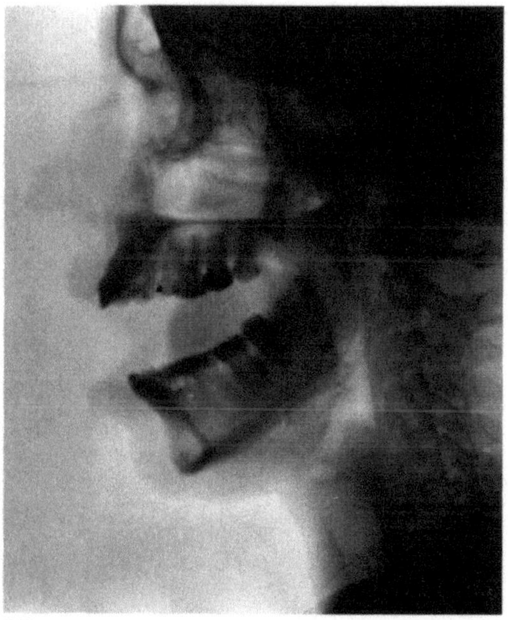

660

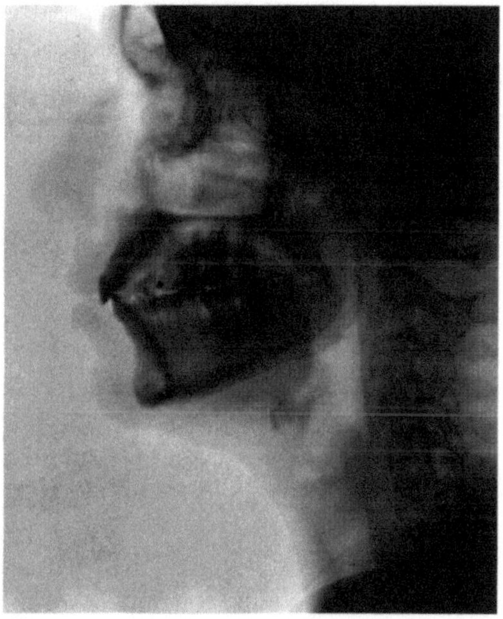

661

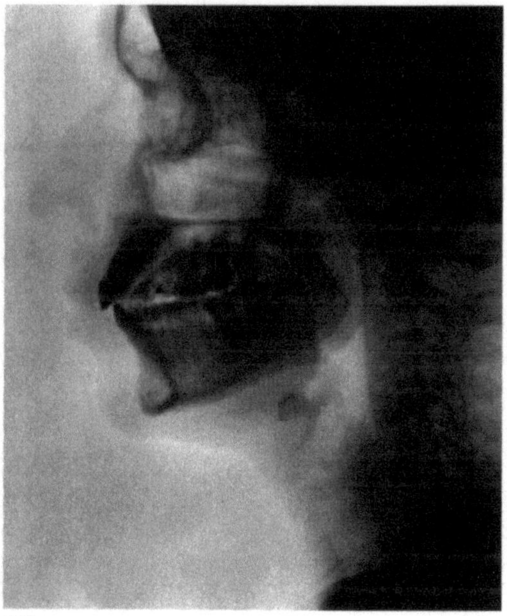

662

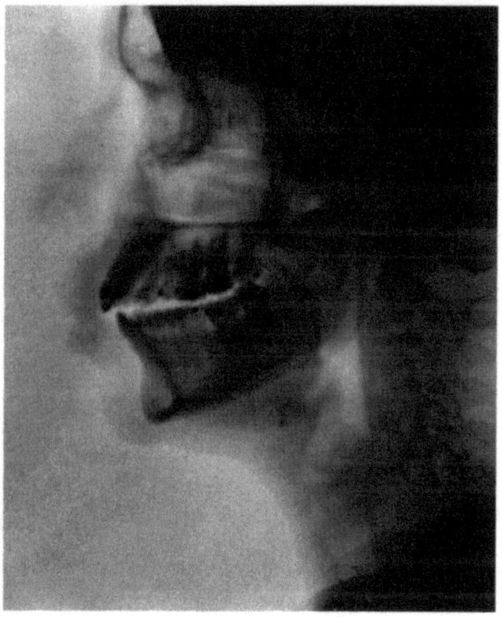

663

661, 662 – speech organs without phonation.
663 – the occlusion of the consonant *b*.

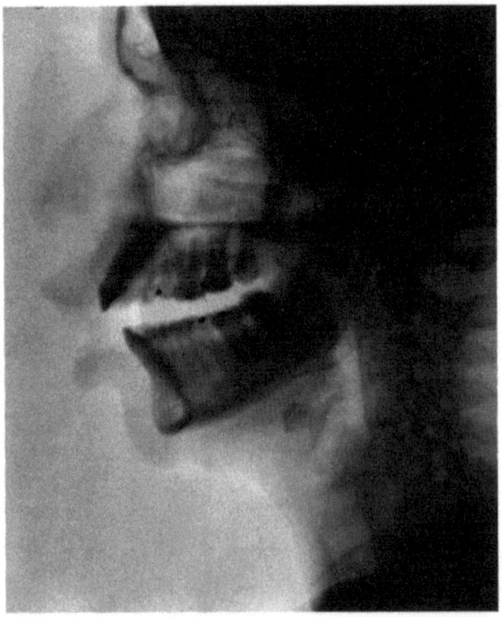
664

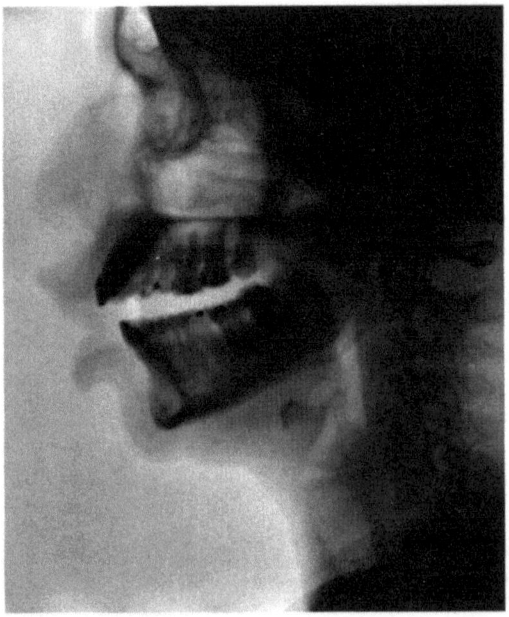
665

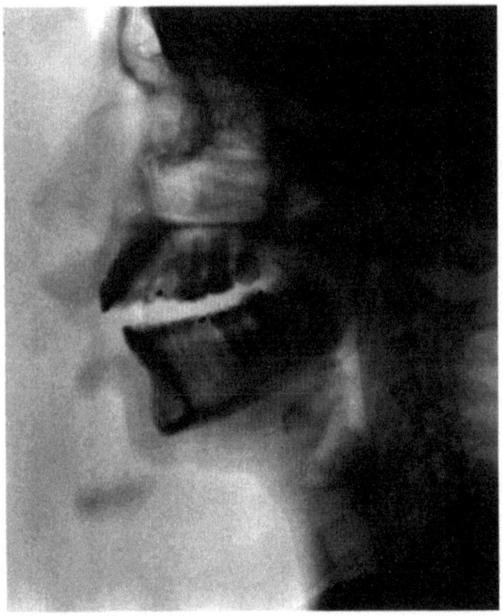
666

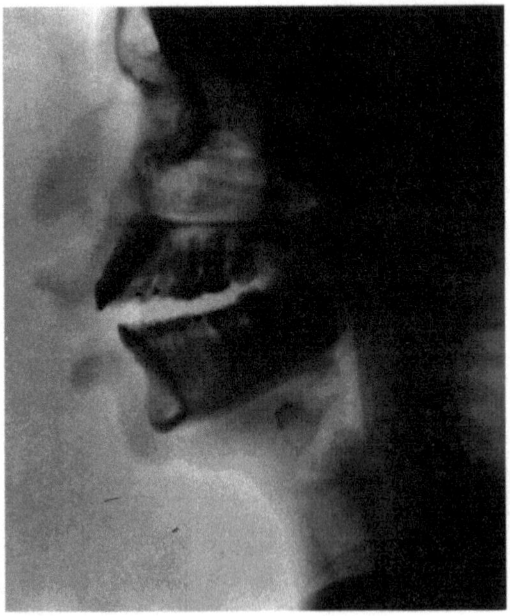
667

664, 665, 666, 667 – the articulatory phases in the singing of the vowel *ó*.

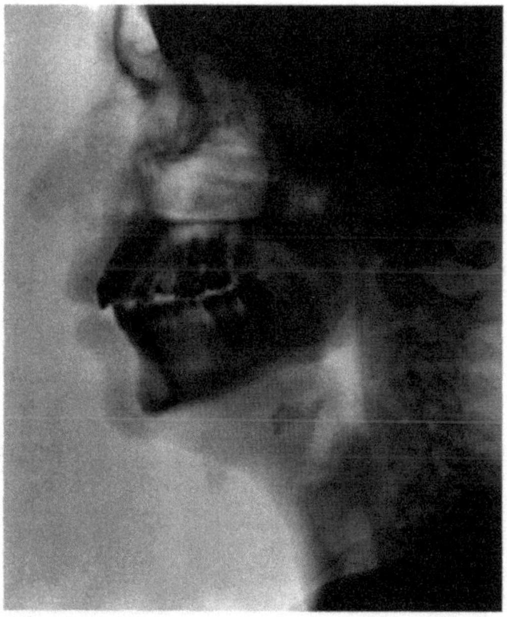

668

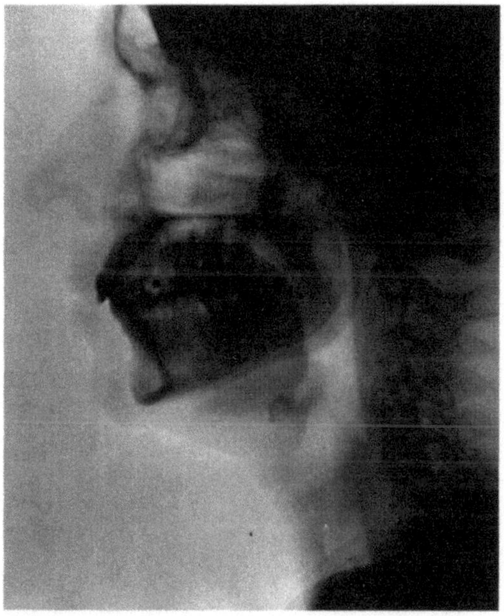

669

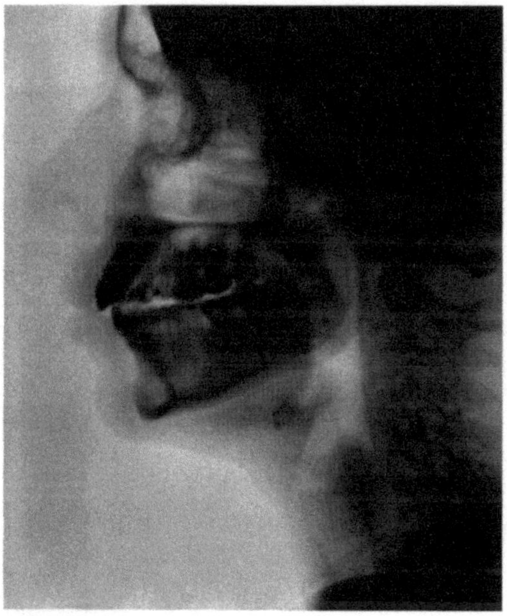

670

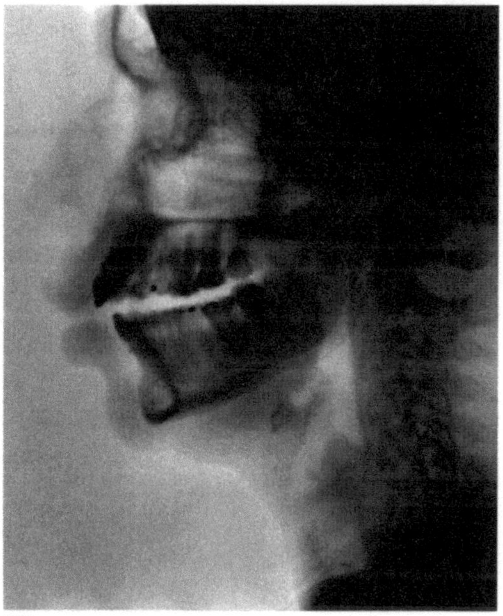

671

668, 669 – speech organs without phonation.
670 – the adjustment of the vocal tract to the occlusion of the consonant *b*.
671 – the occlusion of the consonant *b*.

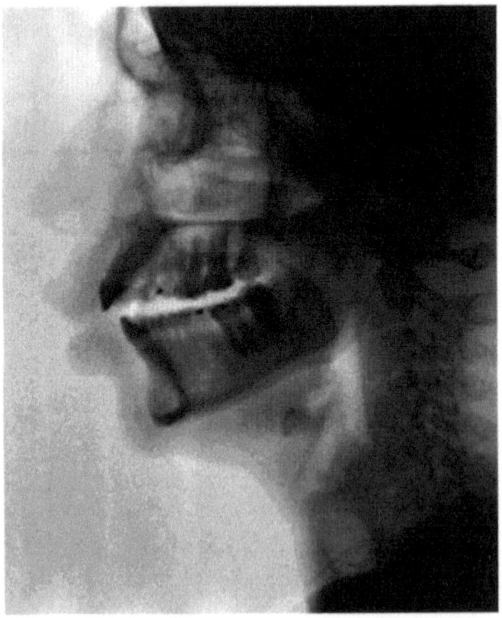
672

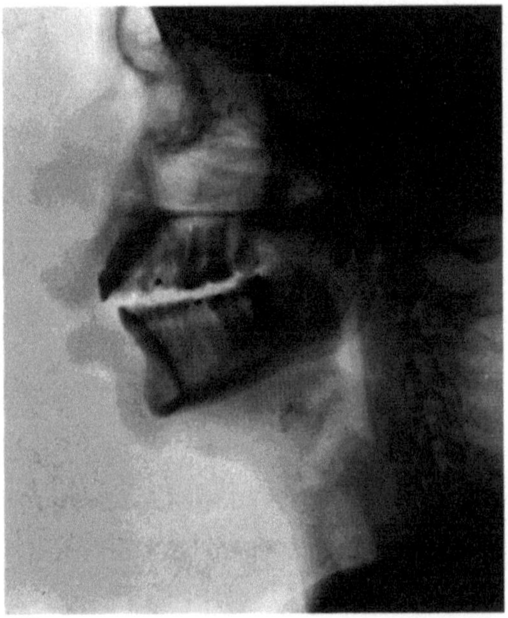
673

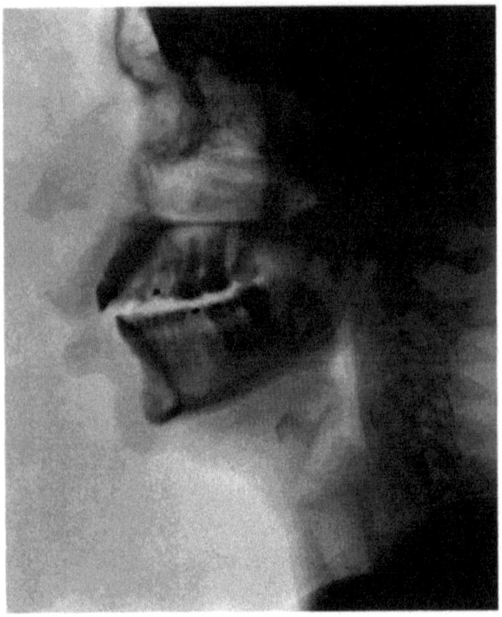
674

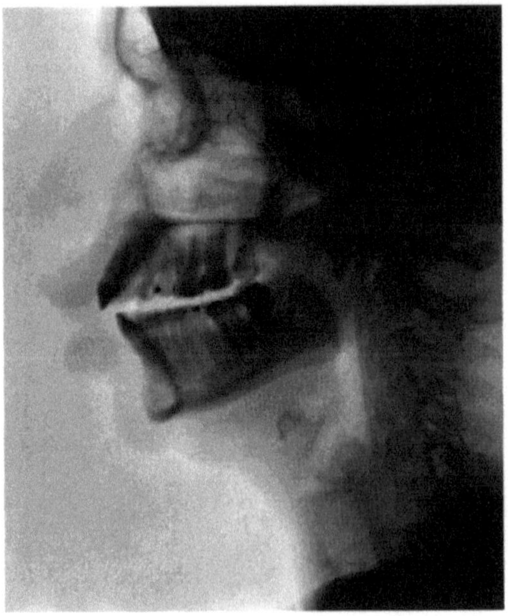
675

672, 673, 674, 675, 676 – the articulatory phases in the singing of the vowel *ú*.

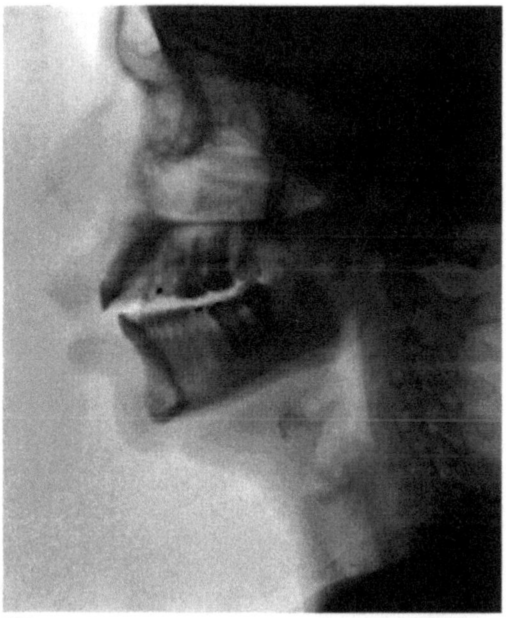
676

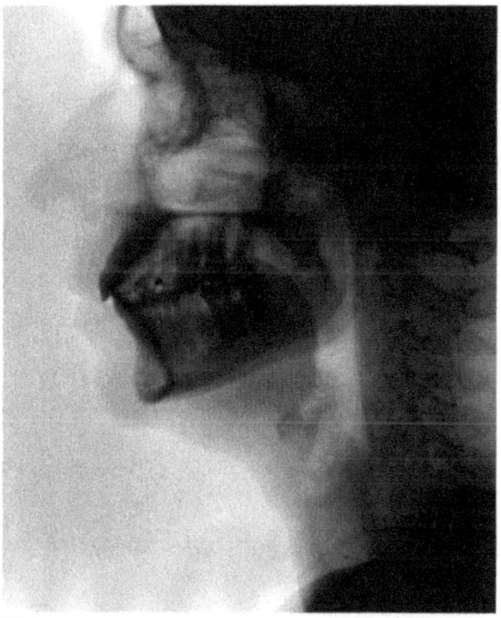
677

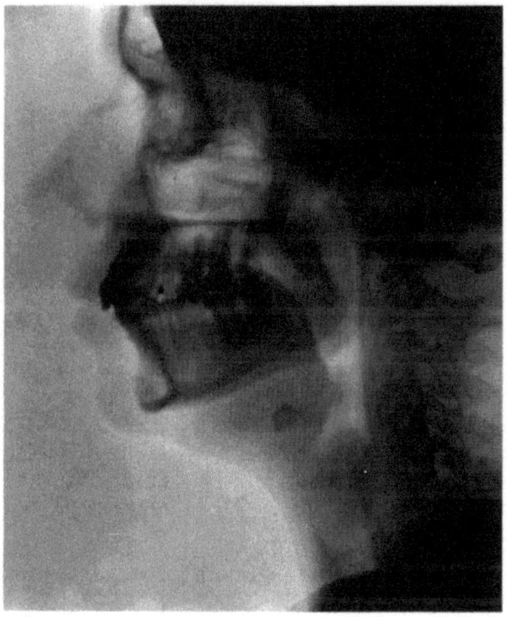
678

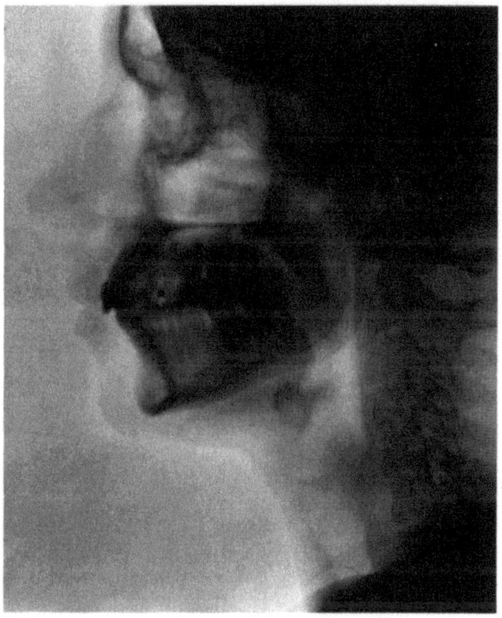
679

677, 678, 679 – speech organs without phonation.

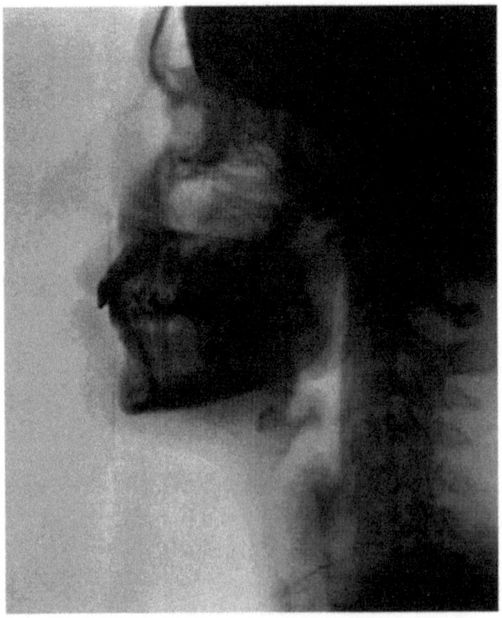

179

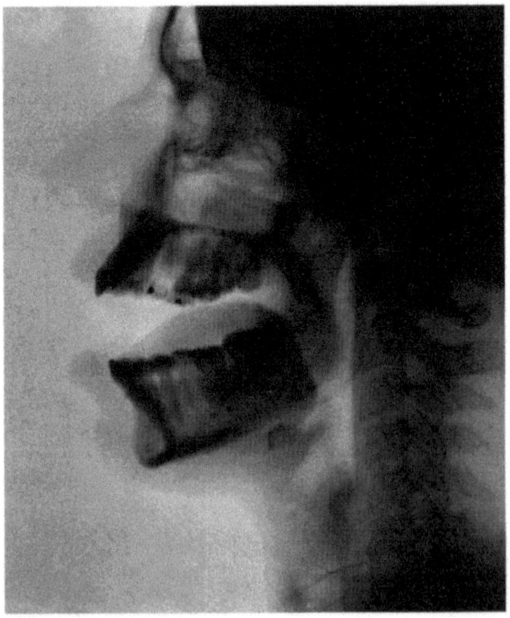

180

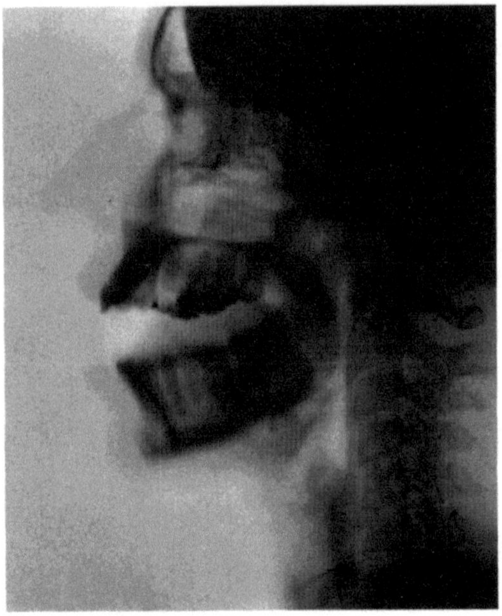

181

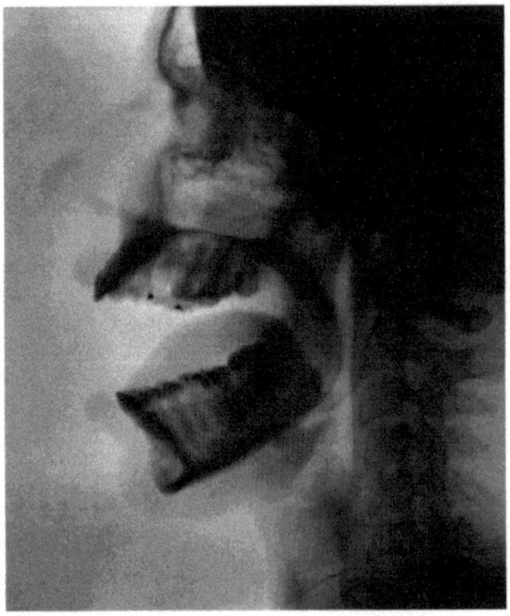

182

Fig. 3 – Pictures obtained by means of serial roentgenography without using any contrast medium. Series No. 3 /HŠ/ demonstrates the speech organs with the mouth held closed and open, during neutral oral and nasal sounds, and during the pronunciation of the spoken syllables *bí*, *bé*, *bá*, *bó*, *bú*. 179 – closed mouth. 180 – open mouth. 181, 182, 183, 184, 185 – the neutral oral sound.

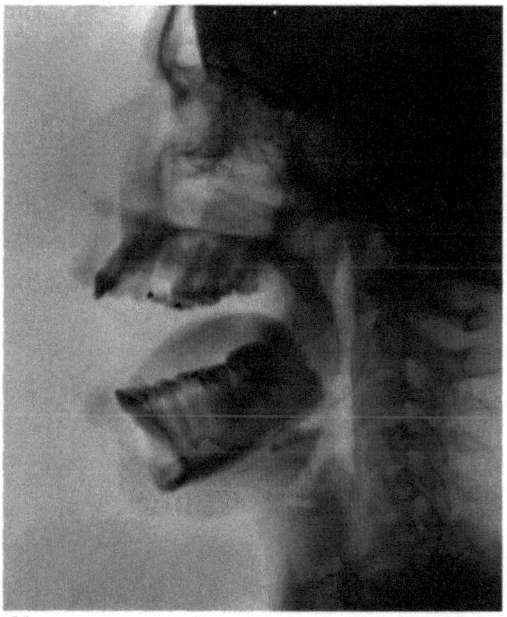

183

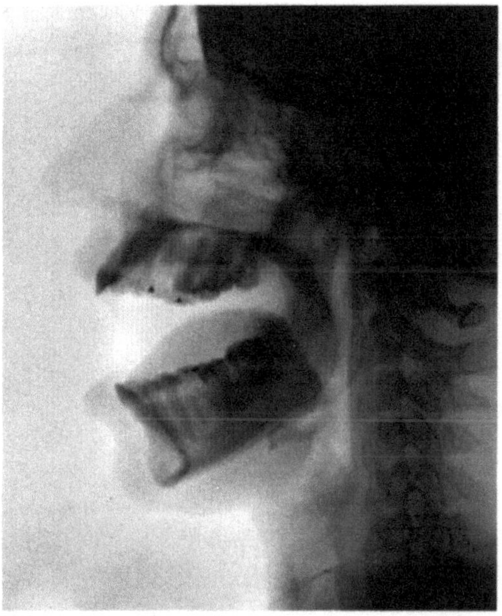

184

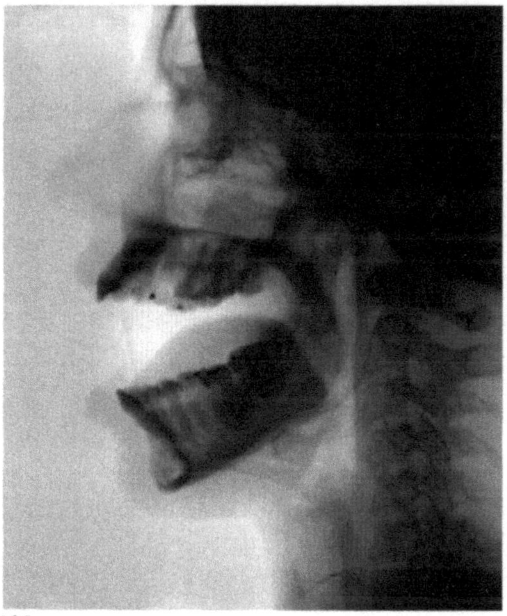

185

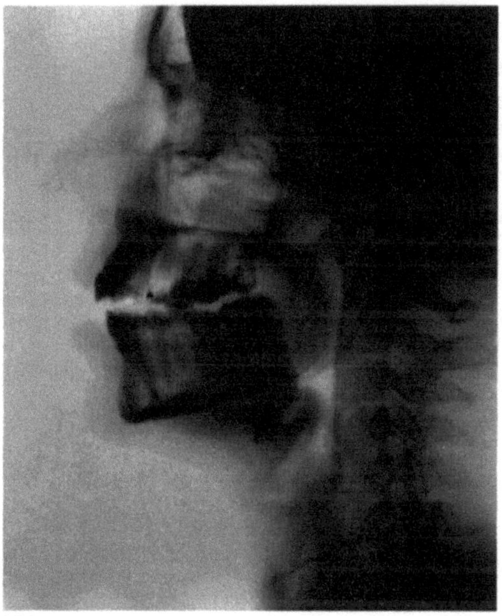

186

186, 187, 188, 189, 190, 191 – the neutral nasal sound.

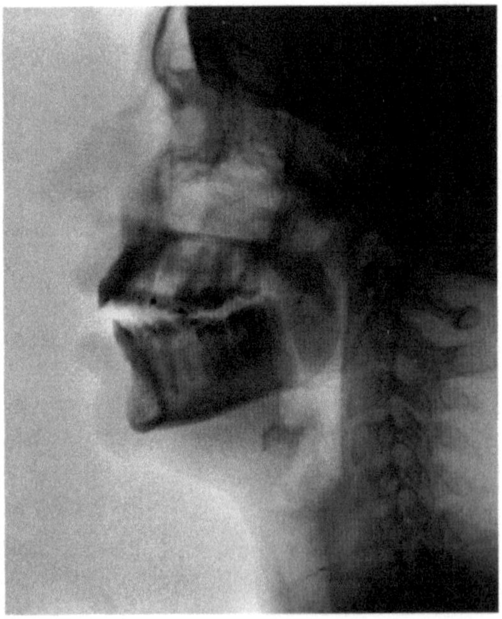
187

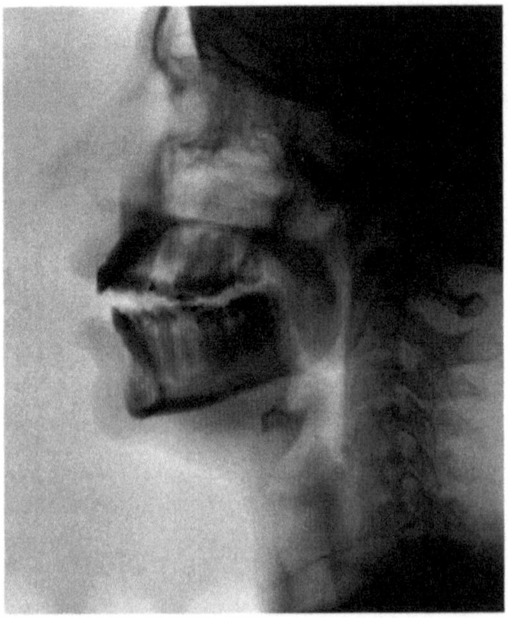
188

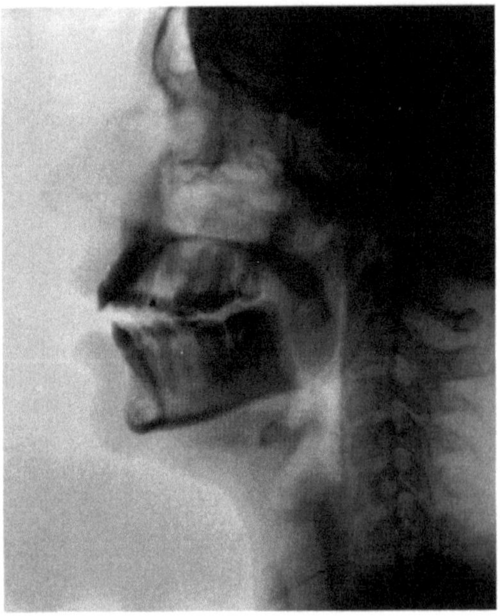
189

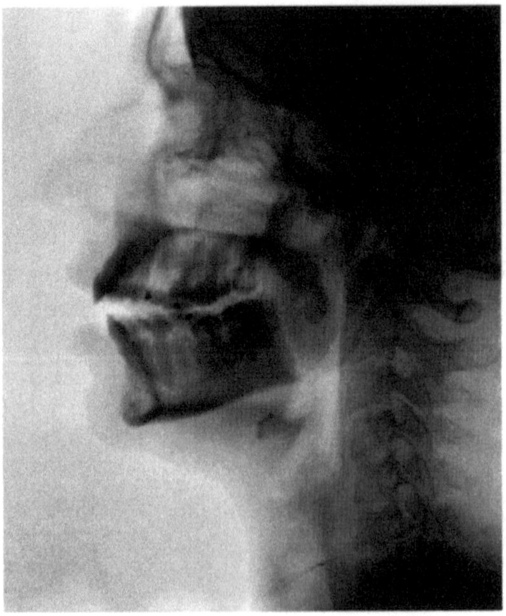
190

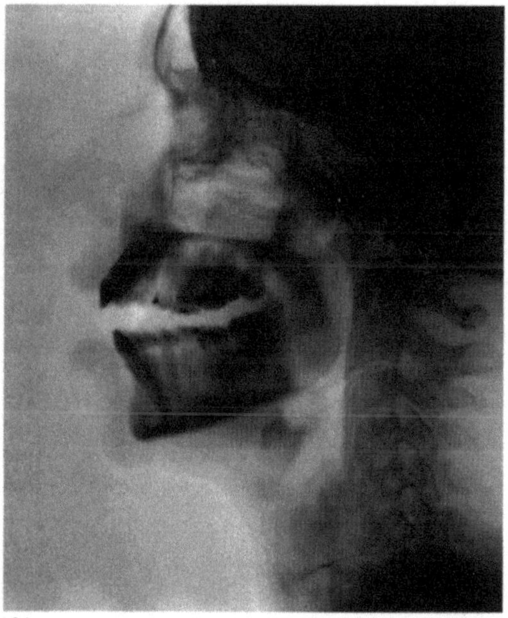
191

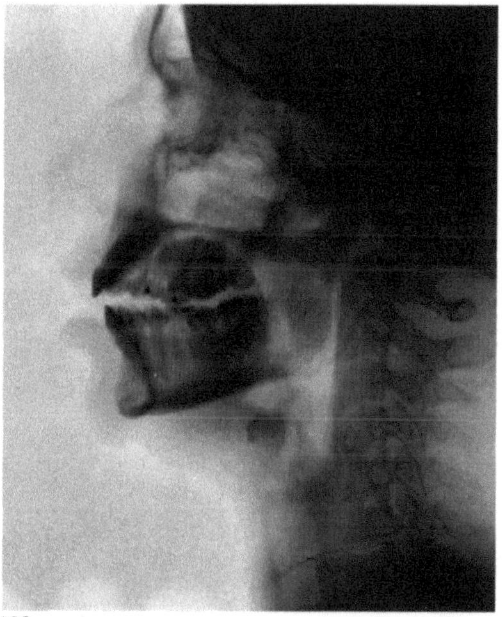
192

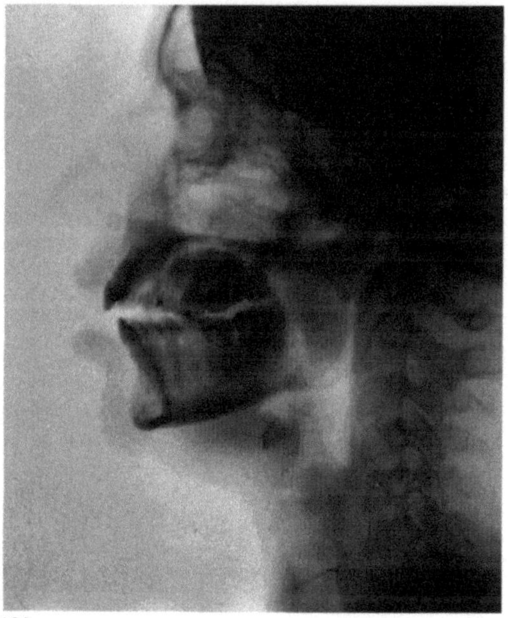
193

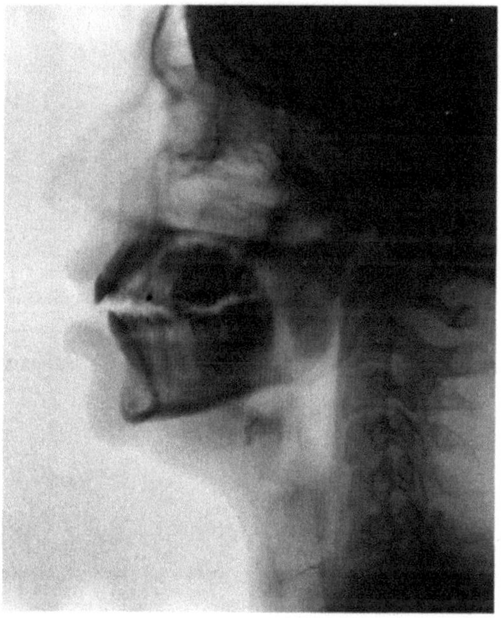
193a

192, 193, 193a, 194 – the articulatory phases in the spoken syllable *bí*.

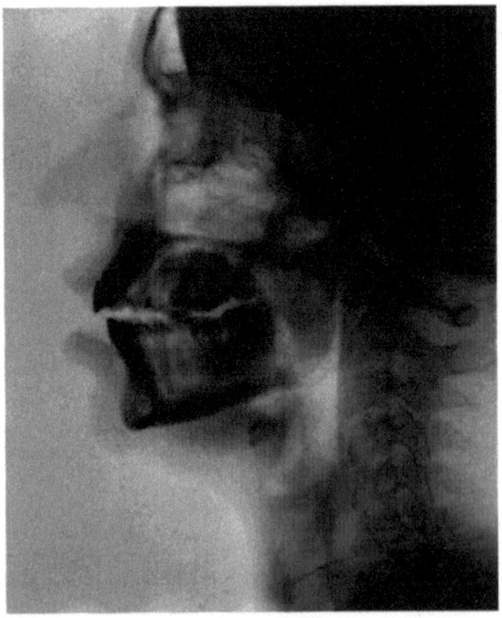

194

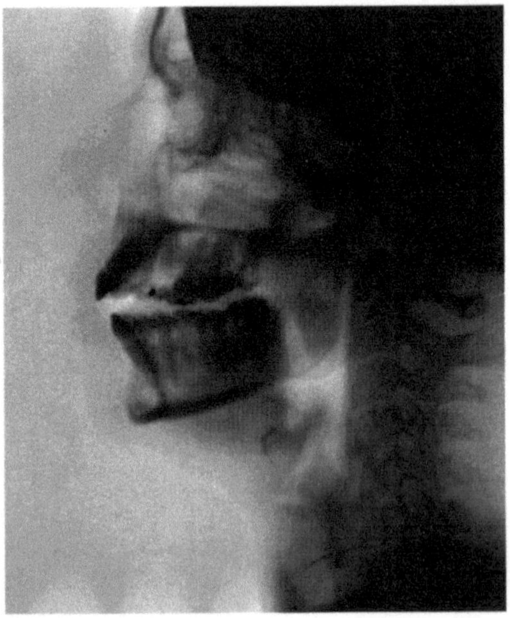

195

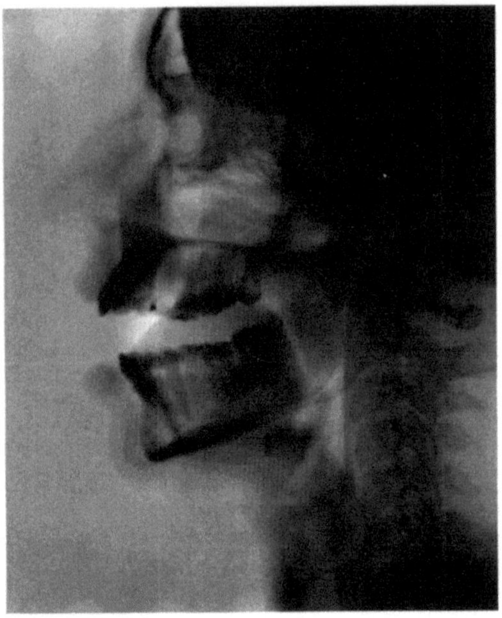

196

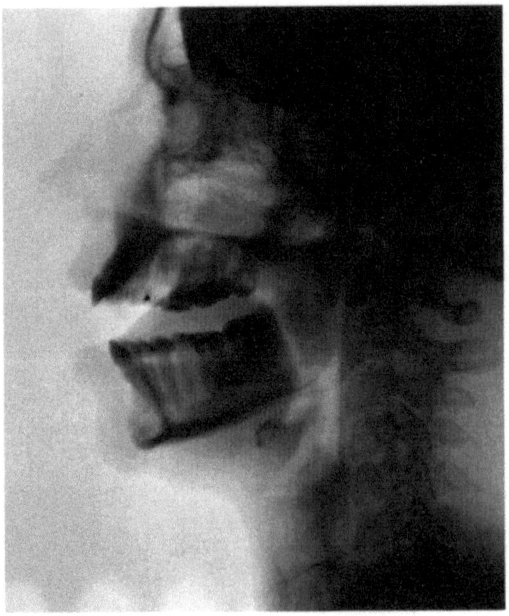

197

195, 196, 197, 198, 199, 200 – the articulatory phases in the spoken syllable *bé*.

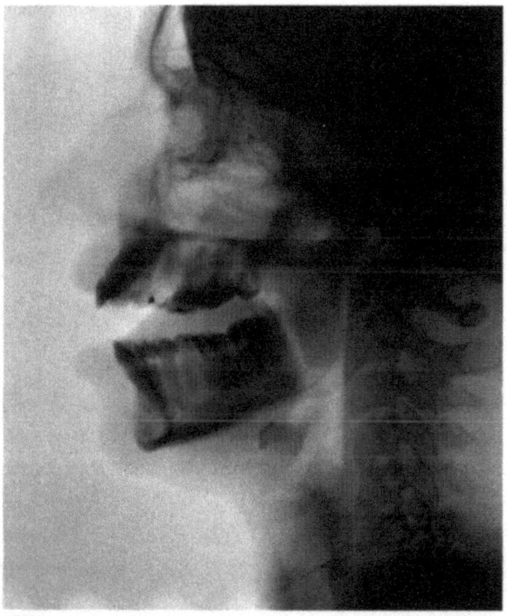

198

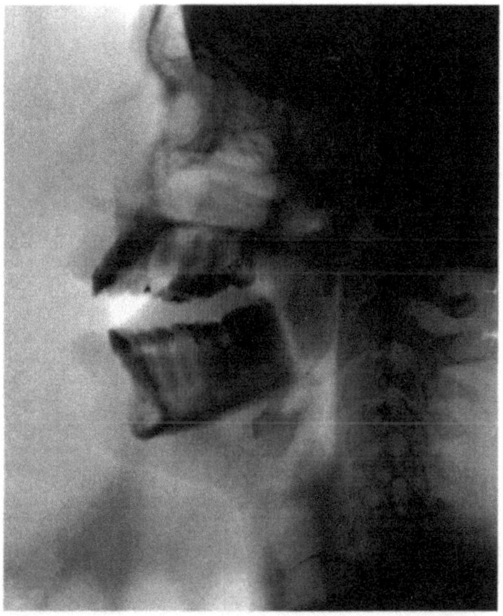

199

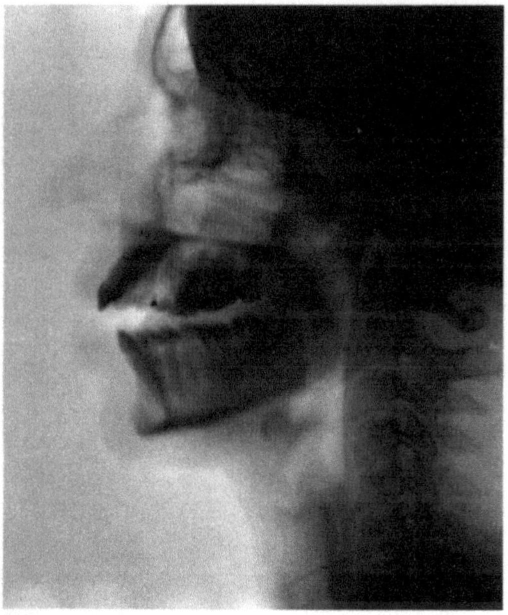

200

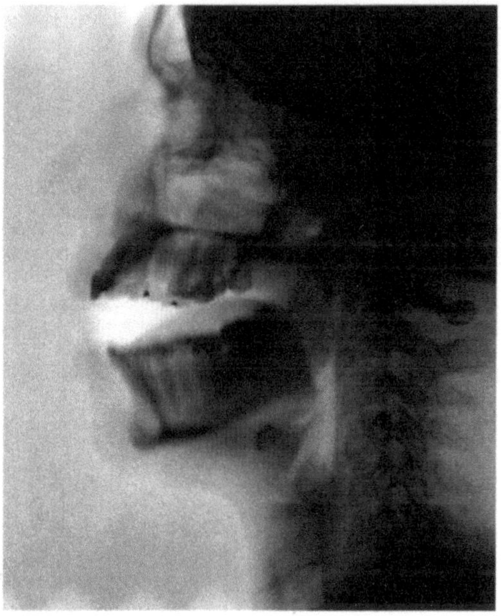

201

201, 202, 203 – the articulatory phases in the spoken syllable *bá*.

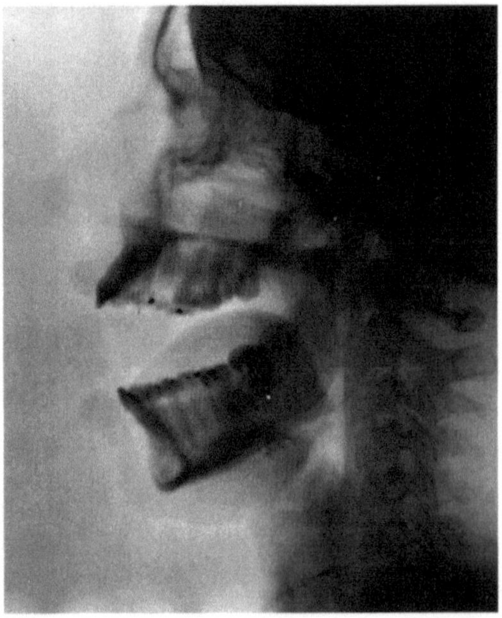
202

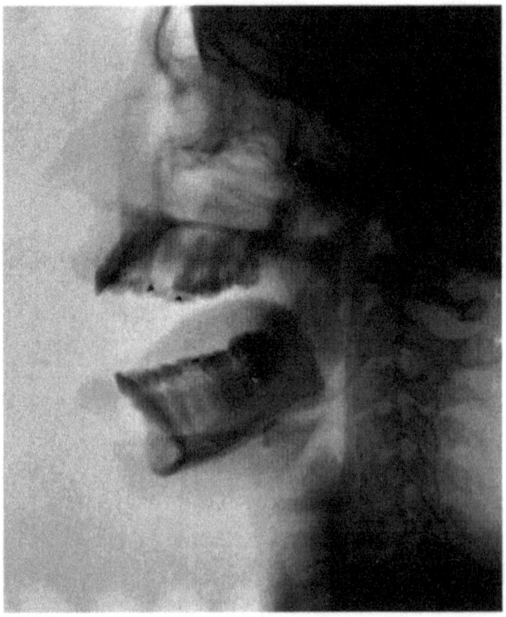
203

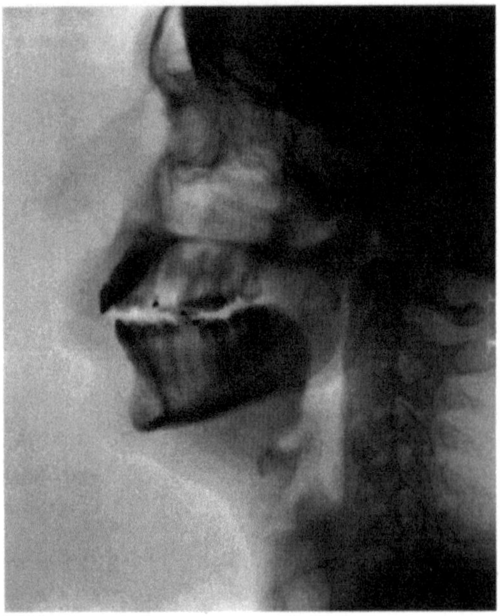
204

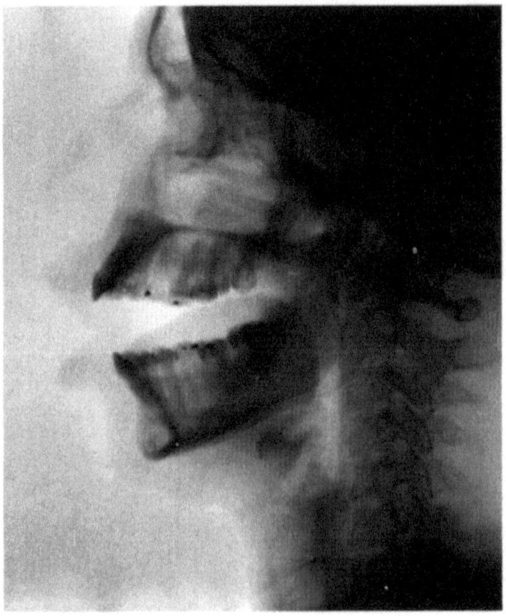
205

204, 205, 206, 207, 208 – the articulatory phases in the spoken syllable *bó*.

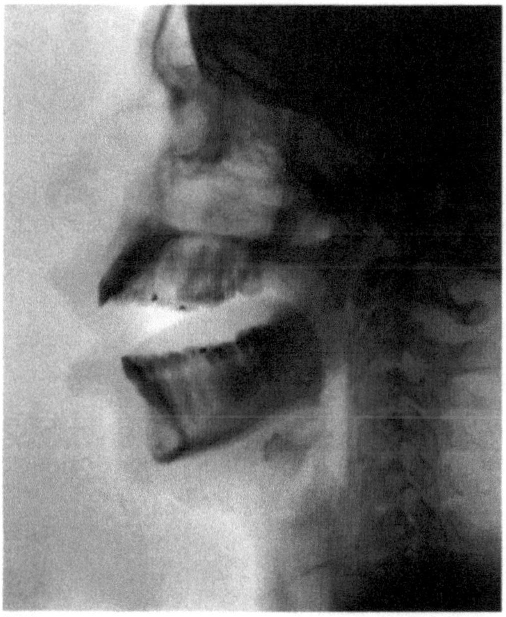

206

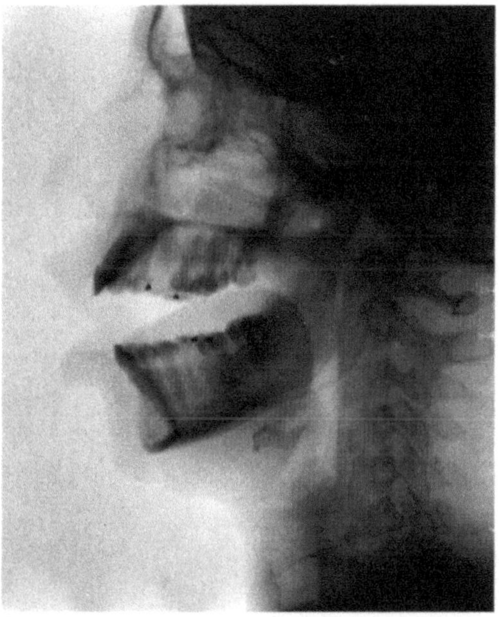

207

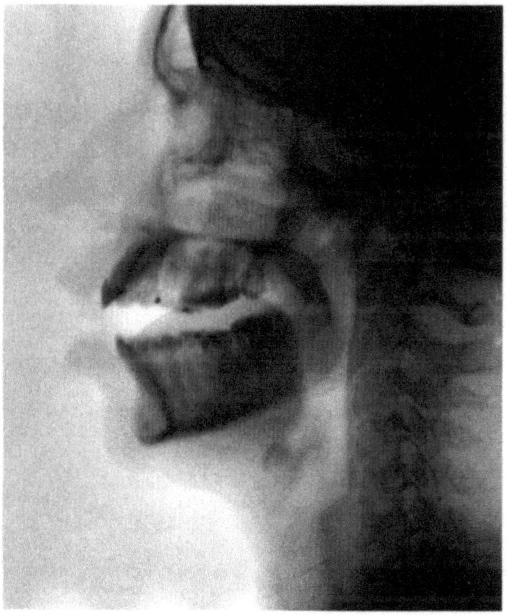

208

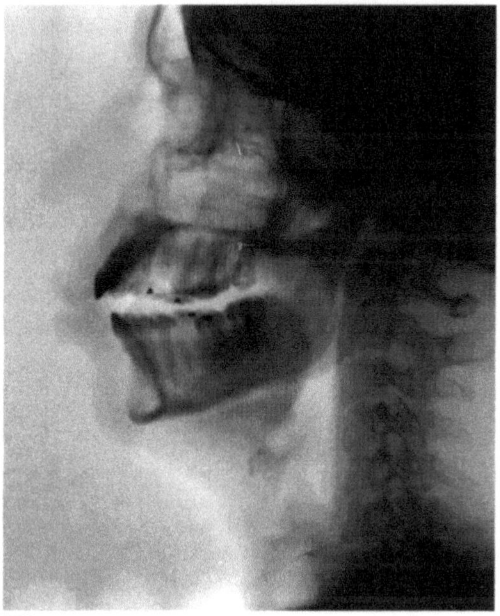

209

209, 210, 211 – the articulatory phases in the spoken syllable *bú*.

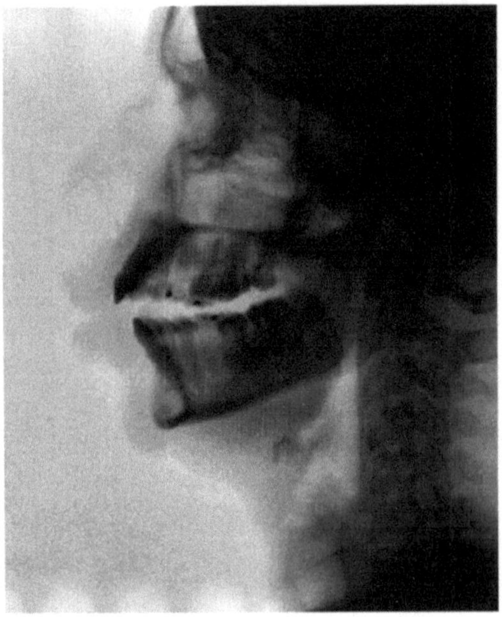
210

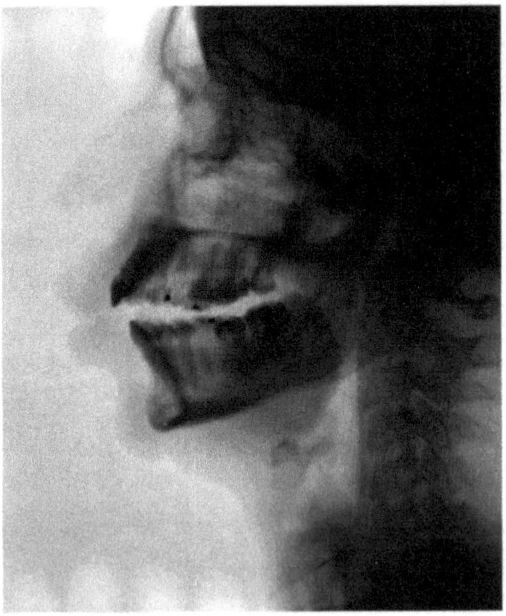
211

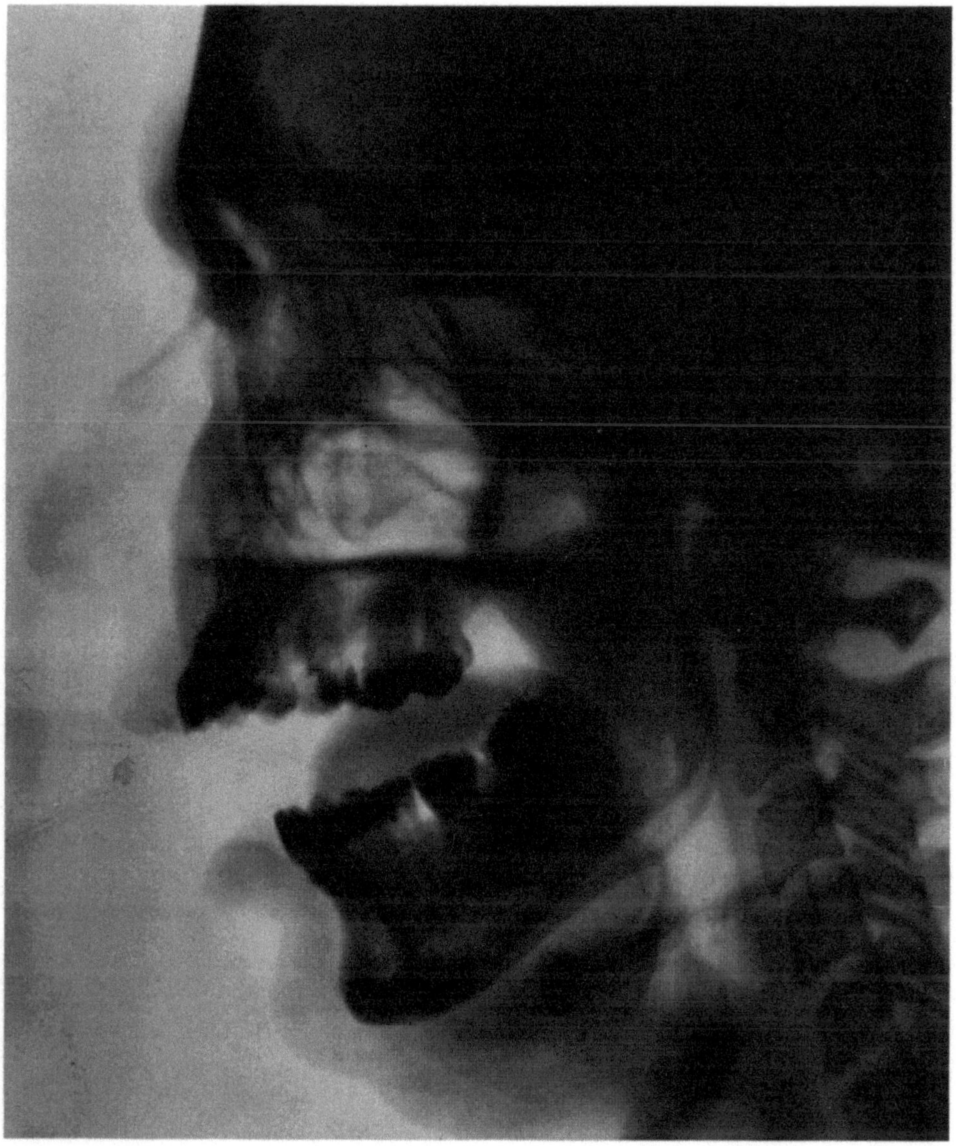

Fig. 4 – The alternation of the velo-pharyngeal closure with the velo-pharyngeal passage during the phonation of sung *é* /series 73–76/.

73 – velo-pharyngeal passage.

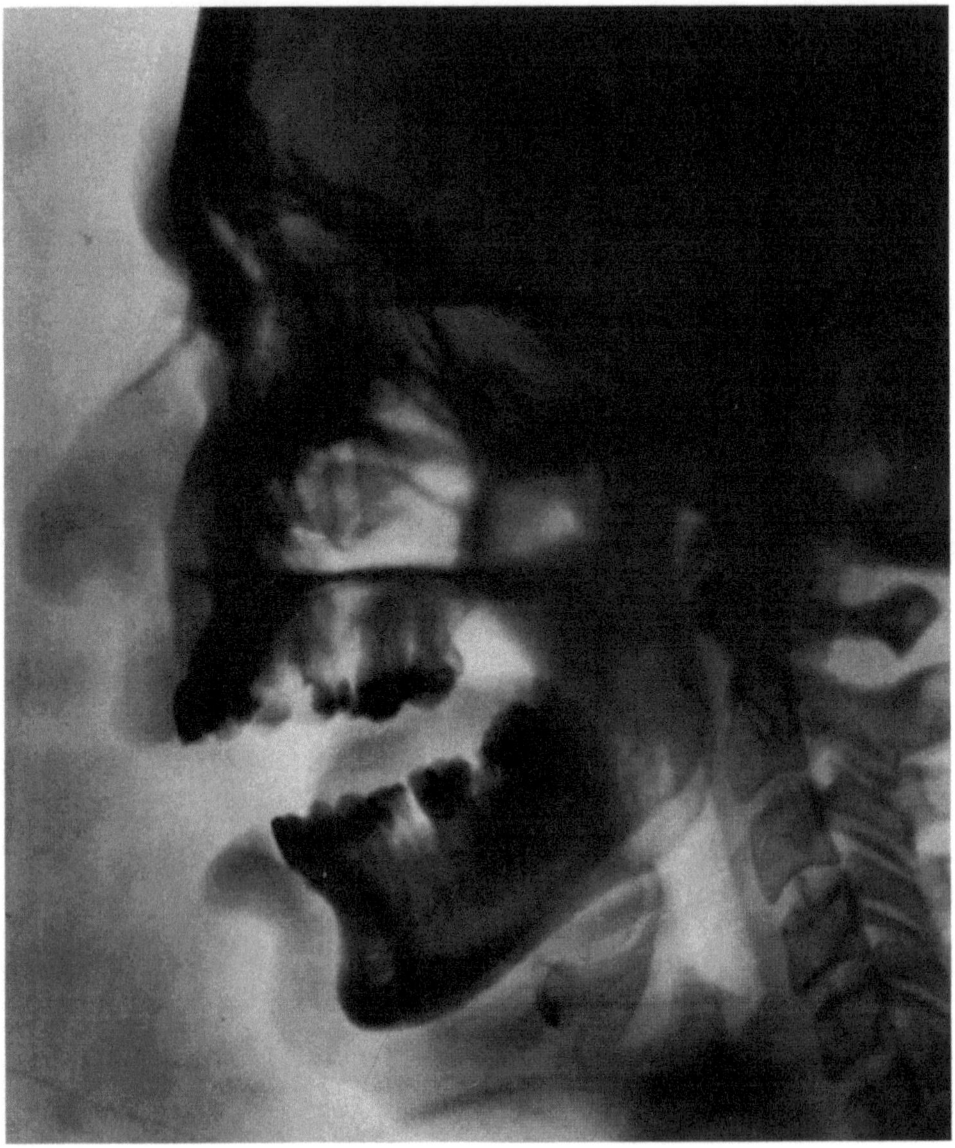

74 – velo-pharyngeal closure.

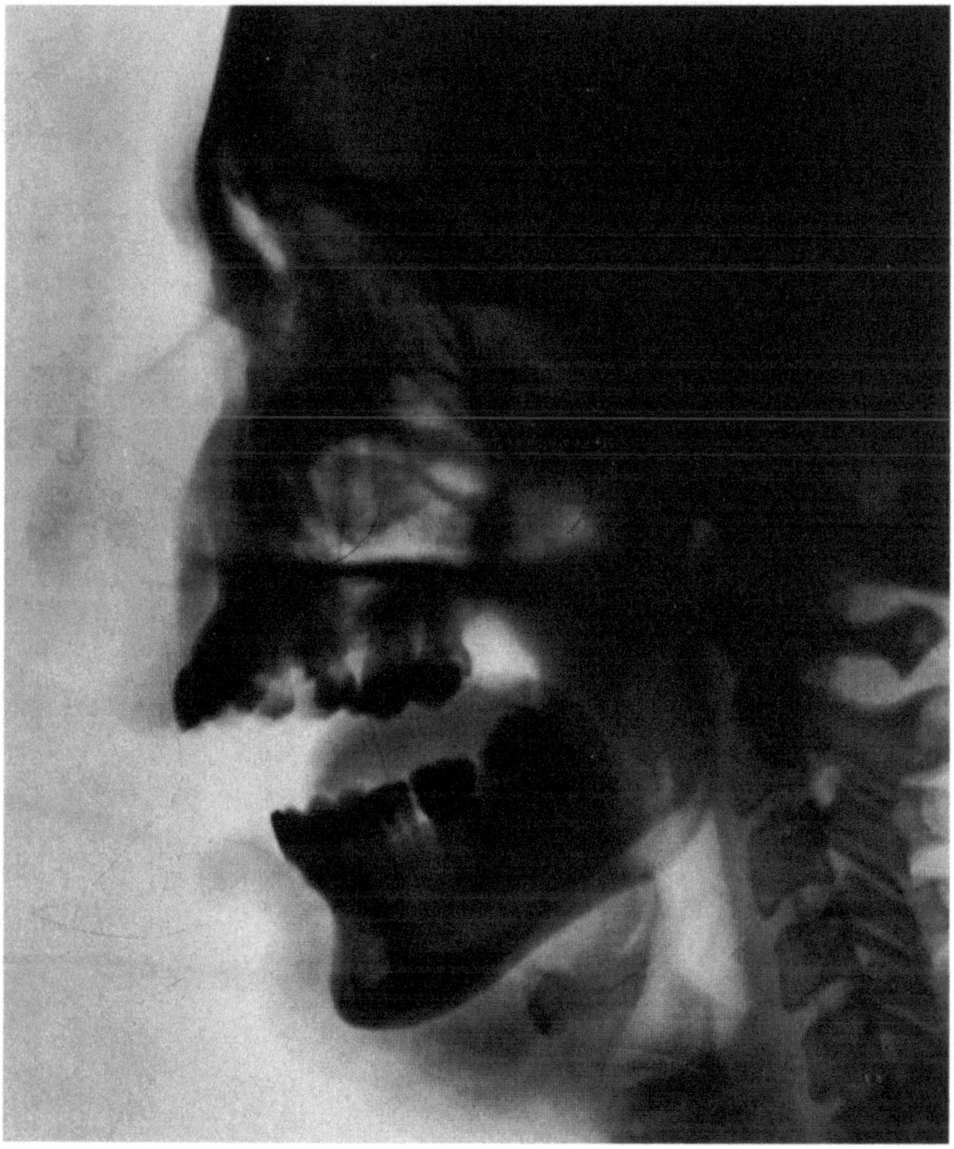

75 – velo-pharyngeal passage.

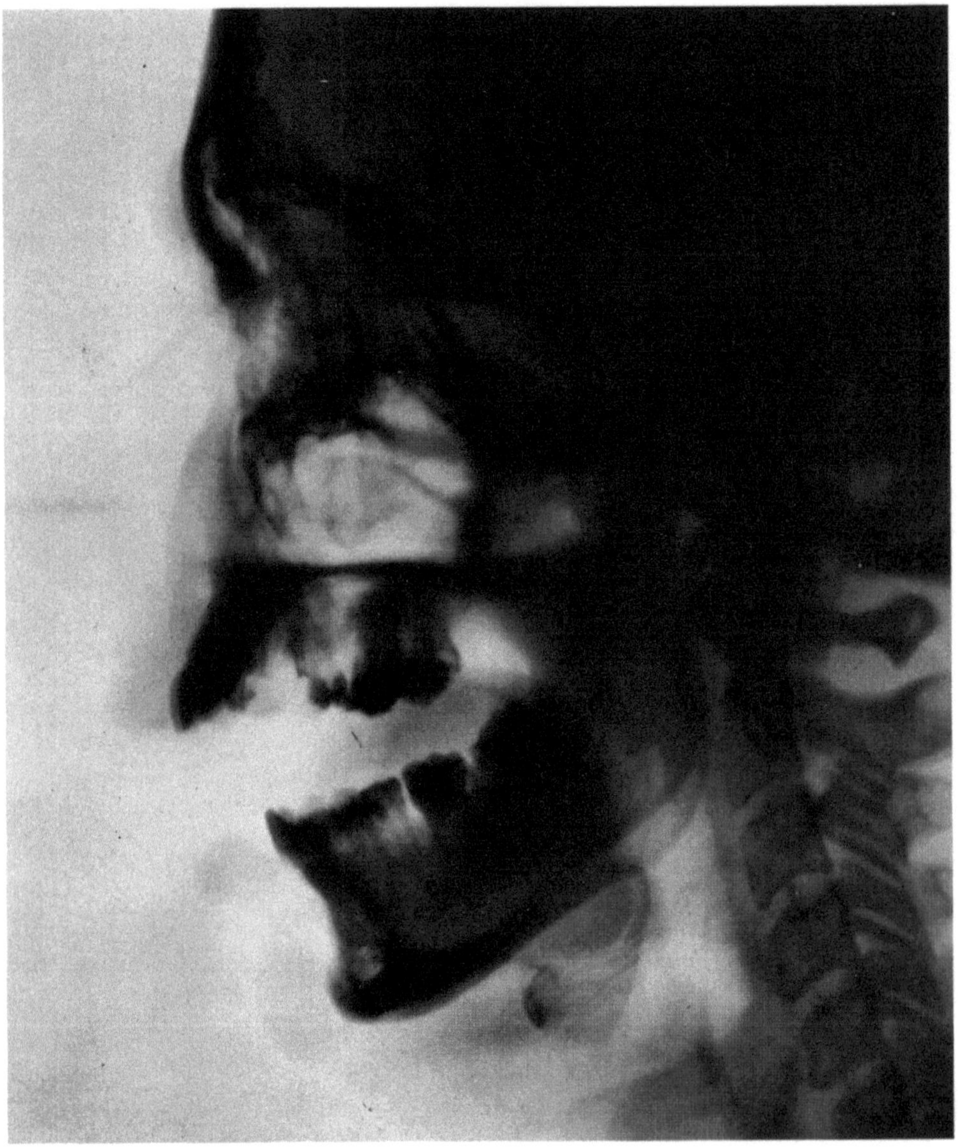

76 – velo-pharyngeal closure.

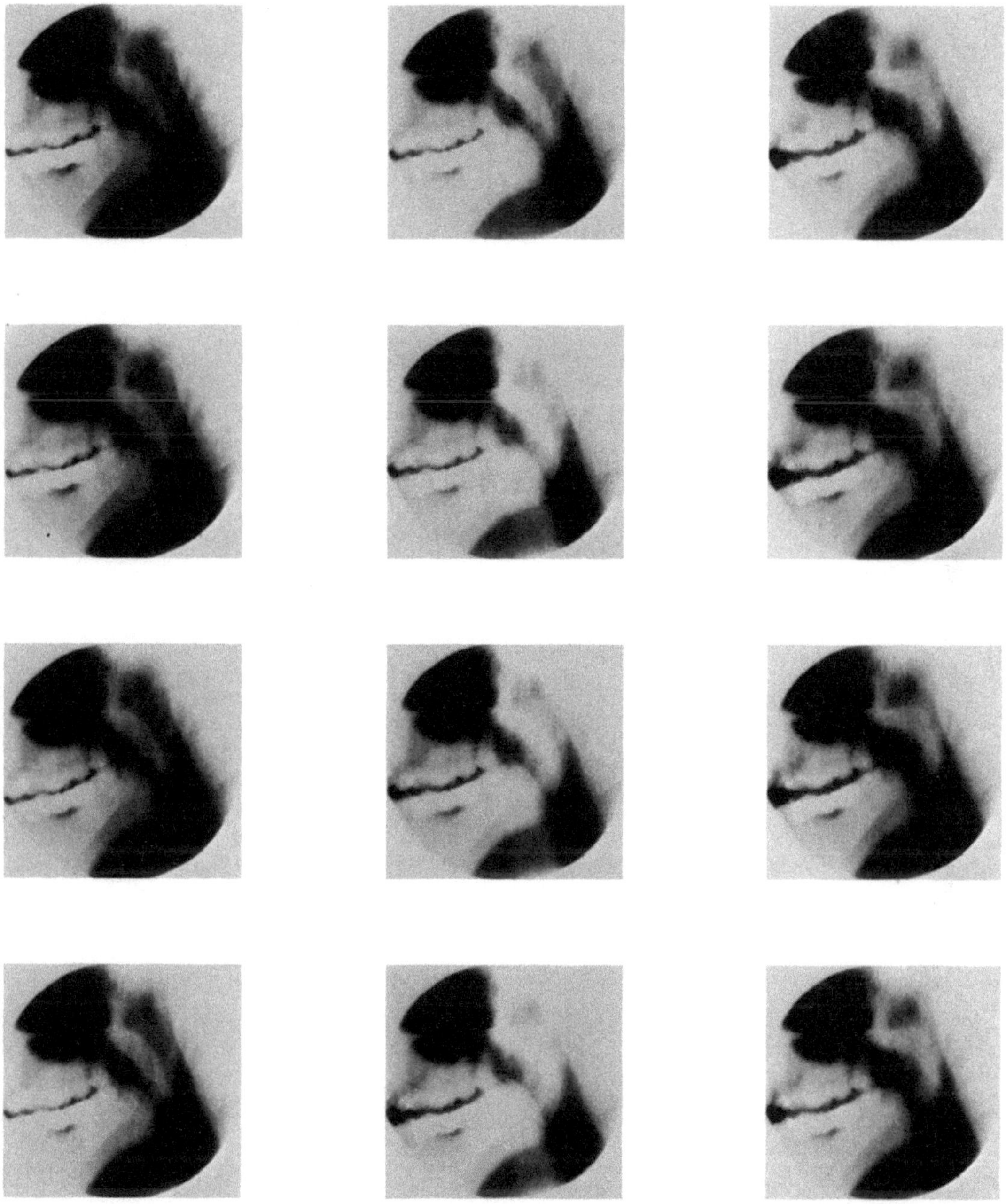

Fig. 5 – Two parts of the cineradiographic shots made during the articulation of the vowel *i* in the syllable *bi*. (The pictures are enlarged; the light parts are dark in the roentgenograms and vice versa.)

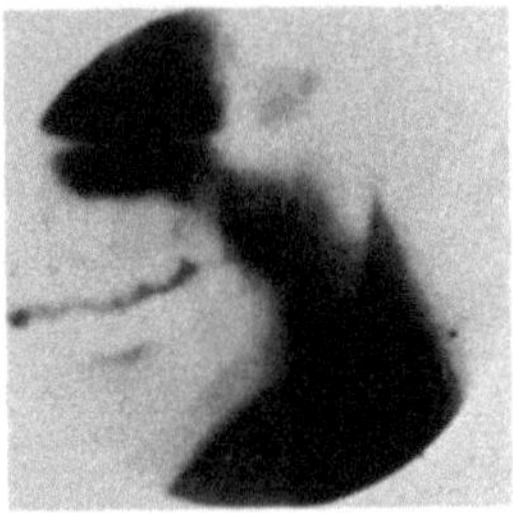
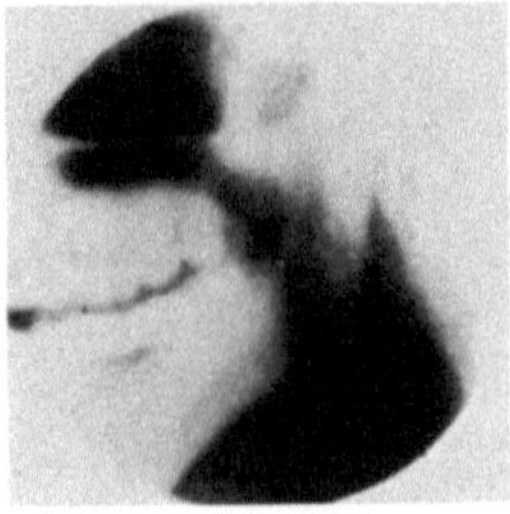
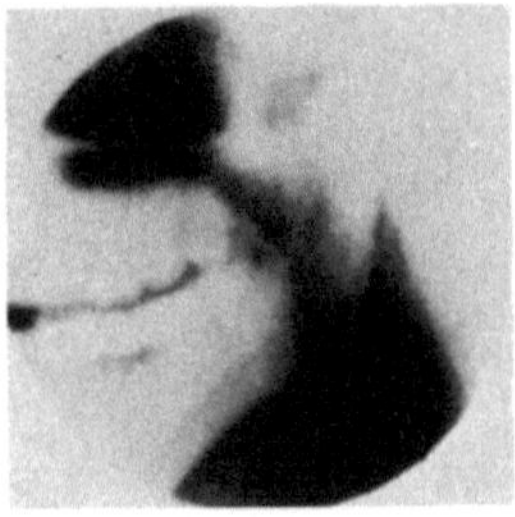

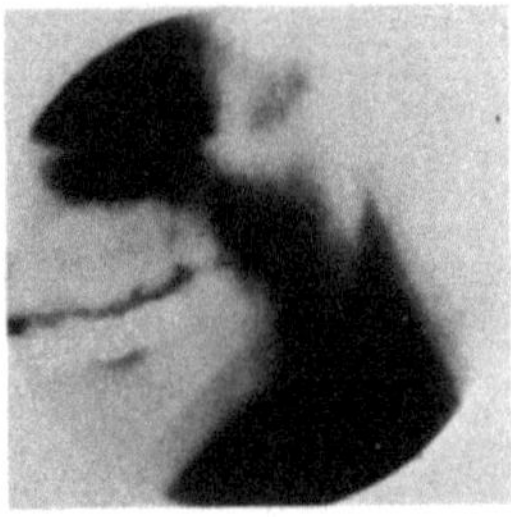
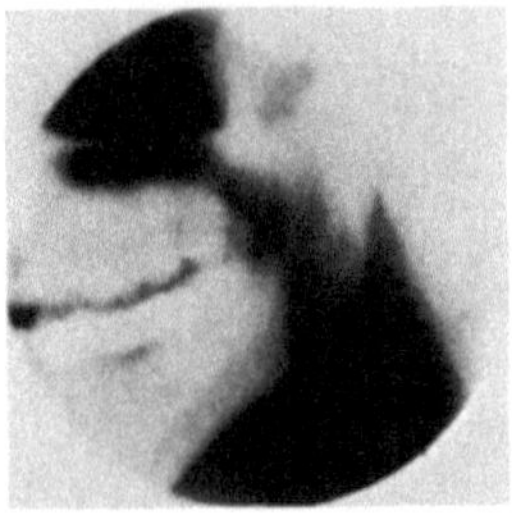
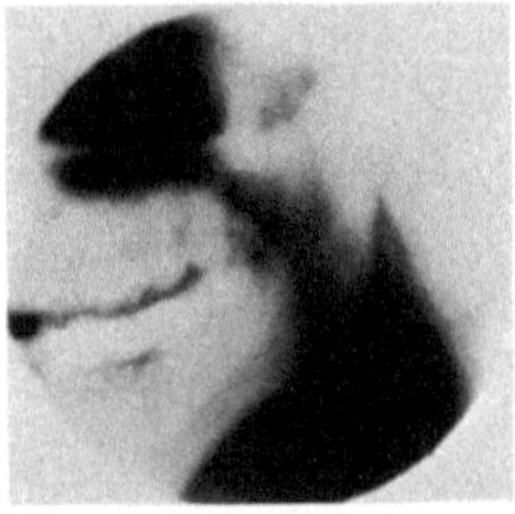

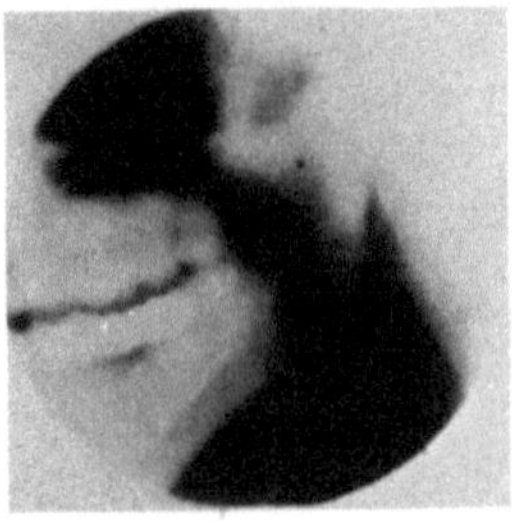
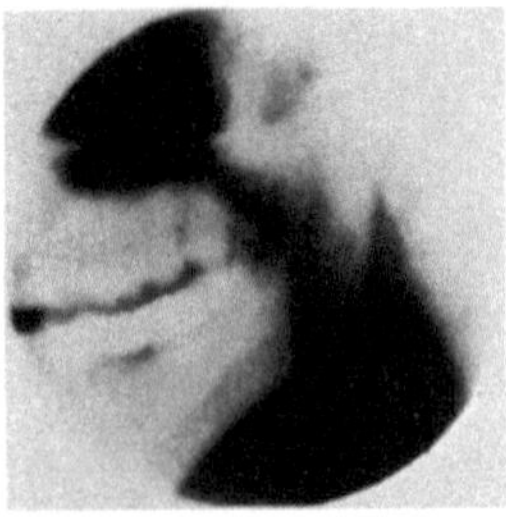
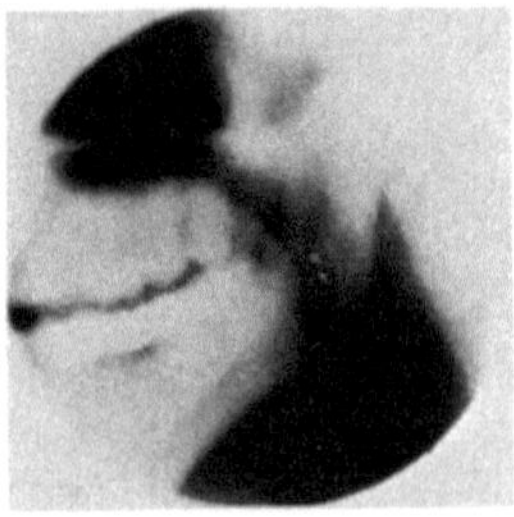

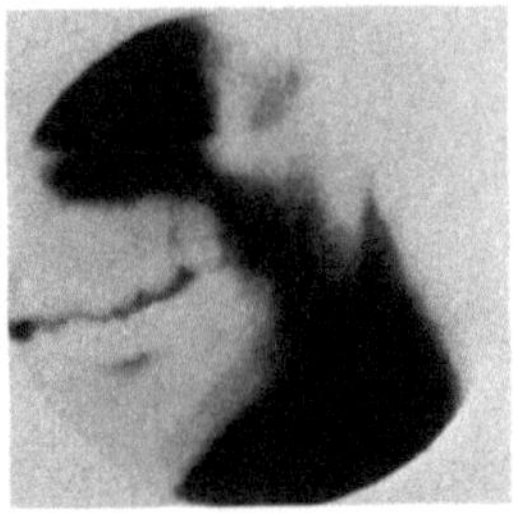
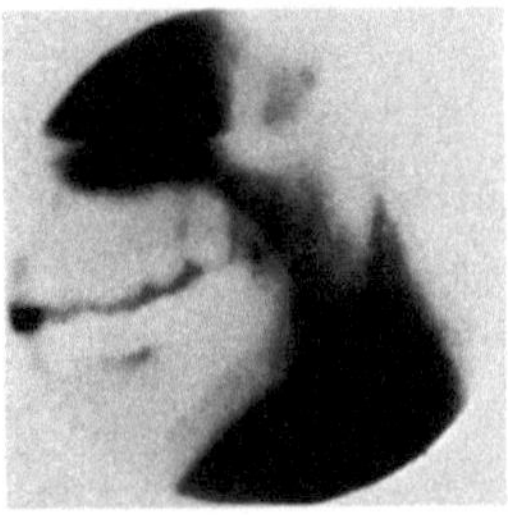
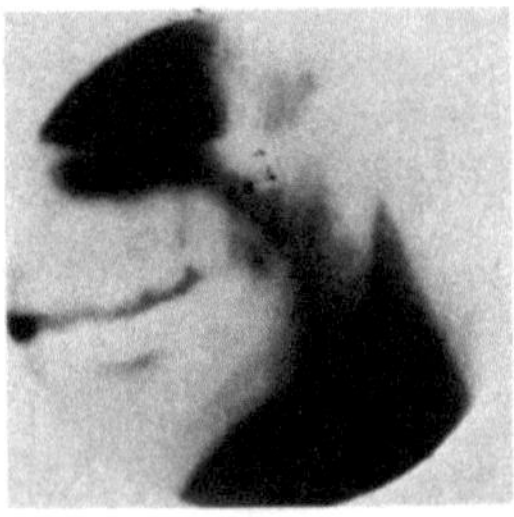

JANUA LINGUARUM

STUDIA MEMORIAE NICOLAI VAN WIJK DEDICATA

Edited by C. H. van Schooneveld

SERIES MAIOR

1. A.J. Greimas (ed.), *Sign, Language, Culture.* 1970. XX + 723 pp. f 140,—

2. Dean Stoddard Worth, *Kamchadal Texts Collected by W. Jochelson.* 1961. 284 pp. f 84,—

5. A.R. Luria, *Traumatic Aphasia: Its Syndromes, Psychology and Treatment.* 1970. 479 pp., many figs. and diagrams. f 96,—

8. Thomas A. Sebeok and Valdis Zep, *Concordance and Thesaurus of Cheremic Poetic Language.* 1961. 259 pp. f 84,—

9. Gustav Herdan, *The Calculus of Linguistic Observations.* 1962. 271 pp., 6 figs., 43 tables. f 66,—

11. Werner Winter (ed.), *Evidence for Laryngeals.* 1965. 271 pp. f 58,—

12. Horace G. Lunt (ed.), *Proceedings of the Ninth International Congress of Linguists. Cambridge, Mass., August 27-31, 1962.* 1964. 1196 pp., plate. f 198,—

13. N.I. Žinkin, *Mechanisms of Speech.* Translated from the Russian. 1968. 475 pp., many figs. f 115,—

14. Ruth Hirsch Weir, *Language in the Crib.* 1970. 2nd. printing. 216 pp. f 38,—

15. Thomas A. Sebeok et al., (eds.), *Approaches to Semiotics: Cultural Anthropology, Education, Linguistics, Psychiatry, Psychology.* 1972. 2nd printing. 294 pp. f 58,—

16. A. Rosetti, *Linguistica.* 1965. 268 pp. f 70,—

17. D.P. Blok (ed.), *Proceedings of the Eighth International Congress of Onomastic Sciences, Amsterdam, 1963* 1966. 667 pp., 23 figs., 2 plates. f 150,—

18. Pierre Delattre, *Studies in French and Comparative Phonetics: Selected Papers in French and English.* 1966. 286 pp., 2 tables, 35 figs. f 68,—

19. Jesse Levitt, *The "Grammaire des Grammaires" of Girault-Duvivier.* 1968. 338 pp. f 74,—

20. William Bright (ed.), *Sociolinguistics: Papers of the UCLA conference on Sociolinguistics.* 1966. 324 pp., figs. f 58,—

21. Joshua A. Fishman et al. (eds.), *Language Loyalty in the United States: The Maintenance and Perpetuation of Non-English Mother Tongues by American Ethnic and Religious Groups.* 1966. 478 pp., figs, tables. f 82,—

22. Allan H. Orrick, *Nordica et Anglica: Studies in Honor of Stefán Einarsson.* 1968. 196 pp. 8 ills. f 55,—

23. Ruth Crymes, *Some Systems of Substitution Correlations in Modern American English.* 1968. 187 pp. f 40,—

24. Kenneth L. Pike, *Language in Relation to a Unified Theory of the Structure of Human Behavior.* Second, revised edition. 1967. 762 pp. f 80,—

25. William Austin (ed.), *Papers in Linguistics in Honor of Léon Dostert.* 1967. 180 pp. f 40,—

26. Robert D. Sutherland, *Language and Levis Carroll.* 1970. 245 pp. f 52,—

27. David Cohen (ed.), *Mélanges Marcel Cohen.* 1970. XXXIX + 461 pp. f 190,—

29. Victor Egon Hanzeli, *Missionary Linguistics in New France: A Study of Seventeenth- and Eighteenth-Century Descriptions of American Indian Languages.* 1969. 141 pp. f 42,—

30. Jitka Štindlova, *Les machines dans la linguistique: colloque international sur la mécanisation et l'automation des recherches linguistiques.* 1968. 336 pp. f 78,—

31-33. *To Honor Roman Jakobson: Essays on the Occasion of his 70th Birthday, 11 October 1966.* 3 vols. 1967. 2464 pp. f 450,—

34. J.C. Heesterman et al. (eds.), *Pratidānam: Indian, Iranian, and Indo-European Studies Presented to Franciscus Bernardus Jacobus Kuipers on his 60th Birthday.* 1968. 654 pp., plates. f 190,—

36. Herbert E. Brekle und Leonhard Lipka, *Wortbildung, Syntax und Morphologie: Festschrift zum 60. Geburtstag von Hans Marchand.* 1968. 250 pp. f 75,—

37. Rudolf P. Botha, *The Function of the Lexicon in Transformational Generative Grammar.* 1968. 368 pp. f 58,—

40. Paul L. Garvin (ed.), *Method and Theory in Linguistics.* 1970. 326 pp. 5 figs., 7 diagrams, 3 tables. f 68,—

41. Johnnye Akin et al. (eds.), *Language Behavior: A Book of Readings in Communication.* 1970. 359 pp. f 63,—

43. Manfred Bierwisch and Karl Erich Heidolph (eds.), *Progress in Linguistics: A Collection of Papers.* 1970. 344 pp., many figs. f 54,—

45. S.K. Šaumjan, *Principles of Structural Linguistics.* Translated from the Russian. 1971. 359 pp., 63 figs., 13 tables. f 80,—

46. Giannoni, Carlo Borraneo (Rice University), *Conventionalism in Logic.* A Study in the Linguistic Foundation of Logical Reasoning. 1971. 157 pp. f 32,—

MOUTON · PUBLISHERS · THE HAGUE

Bei Fragen zur Produktsicherheit wenden Sie sich bitte an:
If you have any questions regarding product safety,
please contact:

Walter de Gruyter GmbH
Genthiner Straße 13
10785 Berlin
productsafety@degruyterbrill.com